How to Eat an Elephant

Simple solutions for lifelong
energy and vitality

How to Eat an Elephant

Simple solutions for lifelong
energy and vitality

Dr Brett Hill

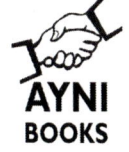

AYNI
BOOKS

Winchester, UK
Washington, USA

First published by Ayni Books, 2012
Ayni Books is an imprint of John Hunt Publishing Ltd., Laurel House, Station Approach,
Alresford, Hants, SO24 9JH, UK
office1@o-books.net
www.o-books.com

For distributor details and how to order please visit the 'Ordering' section on our website.

Text copyright: Brett Hill 2010

ISBN: 978 1 84694 912 8

A CIP catalogue record for this book is available from the British Library.

Design: Stuart Davies

Printed in the UK by CPI Antony Rowe
Printed in the USA by Offset Paperback Mfrs, Inc

We operate a distinctive and ethical publishing philosophy in all
areas of our business, from our global network of authors to
production and worldwide distribution.

INTRODUCTION

How To Eat An Elephant is written for anyone who wants to be healthier. Anyone who wants to make healthy choices but isn't sure how. Anyone who has tried to become healthier and not been as successful as they would have liked. Anyone who is heavier than they would like, isn't as fit as they would like, doesn't have as much energy as they would like, doesn't sleep as they would like, isn't as happy as they would like...

Well, you get the idea: **HOW TO EAT AN ELEPHANT is for everyone!**

Why I wrote the book

When my Year 10 English teacher (I stopped after that year) finds out I have written a book she is going to be dumbfounded. Writing was never my specialty. Ever since I was in early primary school I have always known I wanted to be involved in health care. In Year Two I said I wanted to be a physiotherapist – not too far off. As a result I was always interested in the sciences. I studied biology, chemistry, physics, maths and geography at school. I went on to do a health science degree and eventually a Masters in Chiropractic. Once I left school I never stopped learning and studying. I did some fantastic courses, I went to some awesome seminars and read some amazing books, not to mention having some fantastic mentors, colleagues and mates, and I loved it. The more I learnt the more I wanted to know. In the meantime as I learnt I transformed my health and my life. I was a kid who was sick all of the time, had no muscle mass and a low self-esteem. As a young adult, I thought nothing of a pie, a pasty, a 1.25 litre soft drink and a chocolate bar for lunch, and even less of drinking until I spewed in the evenings. The more I learnt, the more I started to change things and with each little change I noticed improvements, some very slight, some quite dramatic. Bit by bit I got fitter, stronger, healthier, more energetic and by default, more passionate.

After a while though, I started to get a bit frustrated. Not by what I had learnt or by what I was doing but by the fact that no one else was doing it too. I was learning all this amazing information but that information was not getting out to the public. Or when it was getting out it was contradictory, not readily digestible, or didn't explain how to do it effectively. Even my own practice members were having trouble getting their head around it all and learning what they needed to do to get the best results. Fortunately by this time I had met my amazing wife Rebecca, a professional writer with some of Australia's top magazines, and she was able to show me the ropes. What I soon learnt was that writing was easy when you were writing about something you are passionate about.

I have since become much more involved in the media from newspapers and magazines to radio and TV as well as my website www.drbretthill.com and my newsletters. And I have loved sharing my message. What I have found, though, is that often the media only enables me to tell part of the story in small grabs and interviews. What I really wanted to do was show people how to piece the whole thing together, hence my book: the culmination of years of work and study. I hope you enjoy it as much as I have enjoyed the journey.

What is the difference between health care, maintenance care and crisis care?

Well, most of what we currently think of as health care is what I would consider crisis care. Drugs, surgery, alternative therapists and even lifestyle changes can all be forms of crisis care. The idea is that you wait until you have a problem that you can label and then try and do something about it, and the something you do is designed purely to try and remove that label. In other words you have high blood pressure so you take a pill to reduce your blood pressure, you have diabetes so you take medications to try and normalise your blood sugar, you are overweight so you exercise to get your weight down, you have back pain so you see a chiropractor to try and remove the pain. All of these are short-term solutions designed purely to eradicate symptoms. Now there is nothing wrong with that, so long as you understand what you are doing. *It is never going to get you healthy.* In fact that is not even the aim, but it may help to reduce your symptoms – and may even save your life.

I often use the analogy of the oil light in a car. Imagine you are driving along and the oil light comes on in your car. The light is flashing in your face and is really annoying and you want it to go away. Using a crisis care model, you would look for the simplest and easiest way to remove the flashing light. You reach under the dash, find the wire that goes to the light and pull it out. Bingo, the light is out, problem solved and you are on your way. Now of course whilst this is the fastest and easiest way to remove the flashing light, it is not the best idea for your car.

Maintenance care on the other hand is about prevention. It is about attempting to do enough of the right things so that you don't end up needing crisis care. So you might exercise just enough so that you don't become overweight, you may take ongoing medications so that you don't get asthma or you may drink just enough water so that you don't get sick or you may see a chiropractor to prevent your back from hurting. Prevention is always better than cure, so maintenance care is a great way to reduce your risk of needing crisis care, but it still doesn't help you get your body functioning at 100 per cent.

True health (wellness) care, on the other hand, should be about getting your body as healthy as it can be regardless of symptoms or labels or tests. Throughout this book I will refer to this as wellness care because the term 'health' has been corrupted to mean so many different things, many of which have nothing to do with true health. *How To Eat An Elephant* is about eating, thinking and moving as 'well' as you can. Not just so that you don't get sick (maintenance) but so that you perform as close as possible to 100 per cent (wellness). So you eat well because you know that is the fuel your body needs. You exercise regularly because you know it is a requirement for a healthy body. You think positive thoughts because you know they nourish your soul and you see a chiropractor to remove interference from your nervous system because you know that is a vital part of being well. Now of course if you do that, then you will naturally be a healthier weight, you will naturally have more energy and sleep better, you will naturally have less symptoms and you will be much less likely to get sick and therefore need any form of crisis care. *How To Eat An Elephant*, then, is all about simple solutions: so you can gradually and sustainably change your lifestyle to the point where you will have health and wellness that you probably don't even realise is possible.

Think of your body like a car. You might treat your body like a clapped-out old Datsun that gets you from A to B. You use and abuse it and when it breaks down you patch it up and keep on going for as long as you can (crisis care). Of course it won't last as long and it won't drive so well and remember – you can't buy a new body! Or you can think of your body like the family sedan. You know how much you need it and rely on it so you keep it in good shape, service it regularly and keep the water and oil up because you know you can't afford for it to break down (maintenance care). This will keep it on the road, but it is no high performance machine; there is no zing! Or you can treat your body like a high performance machine. You attend to every little detail with the utmost care regardless of whether it is broken or you think it may become broken purely because you want to get the absolute best out of it all the time. You want a long, happy, healthy life full of energy and vitality and you know that taking care of all the little details is the only way to achieve it (wellness care).

Common vs. normal

'But I am not that particular about my body and lifestyle now, and I'm going OK,' I hear people say. You need to be careful how you judge 'going OK'. If that family car was to compare itself to the Datsun it would be going swimmingly, it would probably think it was very healthy and performing fantastically. If, on the other hand, it was to compare itself to the sports car, it would realise it has some work to do. What you need to understand in our modern society is that most people are not well. In fact the vast majority of the western population have some sort of chronic health condition.

Another classic example of Common vs. Normal is ageing. So often I will speak to people and they will tell me a whole list of problems they have and then add, 'But I'm getting on, so it is to be expected'. Often it is not ageing that is at fault, but premature wear and tear caused by poor function or health. For example, people will express to me that their dodgy right knee is a result of getting older. How is the left knee, I ask? 'Well, fine,' they say. And how old is the left knee in relation to the right? They giggle and say it is the same age. So how can it be put down to age alone? Surely if that were the case, both knees would be in strife. Obviously one is wearing quicker than the other and the reason is to do with your lifestyle. It is not functioning as well as it should, so it is wearing and tearing quicker. So be careful of confusing normal ageing with accelerated ageing, and confusing what is *common* with what is *normal*. What is common in our society is for people to be unwell – often remarkably so.

What is normal is a long, happy, healthy life, full of energy and vitality

For some people the idea that this is normal will come as a bit of a shock. It flies in the face of what we see empirically around us all the time. But you need to understand the immense intelligence of your body. Your body is incredibly clever. It knows how to adapt, it knows how to repair and it knows how to regenerate in a remarkable way. Think of the example of a broken leg. I often hear people talking about how 'the doctor fixed my broken leg'. Well, the doctor didn't fix your broken leg. Clever though they are, they could never do something as complicated as mending a broken leg. The doctor may help make sure it is aligned properly and they may give you some pain killers so that it doesn't hurt quite so much (crisis care), but they can never heal the bones. Only your body can do that. Your body can form new bone, new connective tissue, new blood vessels and new skin, all in exactly the right place at exactly the right time. In fact it will do this so well that if you look back at the same piece of bone 18 months later, it will often be stronger than it was in the first place. One of my favourite quotes from a university lecturer of mine was 'the human body is not stranger than we think, it is stranger than we can think', which encapsulates the idea that your body has an incredible ability to heal, the complex nature of which we do not and may not ever fully understand. So if your body is so clever and so good at not just healing from injury and trauma, but also staying healthy, then why are so many people so sick?

It's not our bodies that are sick, it's our environments
Our bodies have evolved over millions of years to be and stay well. The only problem is that the world they were designed for has changed dramatically. It has been shown that our genes have changed very little in the last 100,000 years, but think how much our environment has changed in that time – from hunter gatherers who exercised daily, only ate fresh real foods and had a supportive community environment to our modern world of concrete jungles, sitting all day, repetitive activities, junk food and stress! This has all changed in such a remarkably short period of time that our bodies have not had a chance to adapt. I mean, if the genes have barely changed in 100,000 years, how could we be expected to adapt to the immense change that has

happened in the last 100 years alone?

A classic example of the way our bodies have not adapted to our modern environment is our stress response. We were originally designed for the kinds of stressors our hunter gatherer ancestors had: short-lived intense stress, like running from a mammoth or fighting with a spear. Our stress response contains many clever adaptations. In order to help us 'fight or flight', our blood pressure is raised, we pump more sugar and fat into our blood stream for energy, our blood vessels constrict, our clotting factors increase in case we bleed, our senses are heightened, we become anxious and we switch off all of the things that don't help us fight or flight (like cellular immunity, memory and concentration, digestion, sex drive, growth and bone density). All of this makes sense for a hunter gatherer who is fighting or running. Translate it into our modern world, though, and you start to see an alarming picture.

Our modern lifestyles are full of chronic stressors rather than acute ones. We tend to be stressed all the time as a result of work pressures, money pressures, family pressure etc. This means that many people's stress response is permanently switched on. Have a look back at that list and see what is always switched on and what is off. You will see an alarming correlation between the list and the chronic lifestyle diseases that plague our western societies. High blood pressure, blood vessel constriction and excess fat in the blood stream and increased blood clotting factors are a recipe for heart disease. Excessive sugar in the blood stream and increased insulin resistance in the cells is a recipe for diabetes. Decreased cellular immunity puts you at increased risk of many diseases including cancer, and I could go on and on. The point I am getting at here, though, is that the response from our bodies is actually very intelligent. In fact if we had not created such an unhealthy environment around ourselves, it would be exactly what our bodies need to get and stay well, each and every time. So what needs to change is the environment we are putting ourselves in.

So whose fault is it that we are all so sick?

So often we want to blame everyone else for our health problems. Wellness expert Dr James Chestnut says that we tend to blame our health on "bad luck, bad germs or bad genes". We know that our genes have not changed, we also know that most of our modern chronic diseases (like heart disease and diabetes) have nothing to do with germs and we know there is more to it than just dumb luck. But if we are not blaming germs, genes or luck then we need someone to blame, right? So we start to blame the government for not regulating against it, or we blame super-markets for not giving us healthy options, or we blame fast food outlets for not serving healthier options, or we blame pharmaceutical companies for only selling quick fixes. In reality, though, the blame lies a lot closer to home. It is you who is in control of your health. It is you who decides what goes in your mouth, it is you who decides whether and how you exercise, and it is you who controls your thoughts (yes really). So it is time to step up to the plate and start taking charge of your health.

So how do I know if I'm healthy?

OK so if we can't use how we feel to measure how healthy we are then how do we know if we are healthy? Well we could go into the Doctor and run a whole series of tests. We could do a blood test to check our body chemistry, we could take our blood pressure, we could get our blood sugar levels checked. The problem is we all know stories of people who were 'given the all clear' by their Doctors only to be struck down by illness later on. The problem is that the tests we do are only as good as the current level of understanding of the body, and there is still a lot we don't know. The other issue with this approach is that whilst it may allow us to catch a problem early is does not allow us to prevent it. These markers of ill health only present once the problem is established. Perhaps the best way then to measure your level of health is to look at what you do. Do what I call a health audit and really honestly analyse what you are eating, what sort of thoughts you think on a day to day basis and what sort of exercise you are getting into your weekly routine. Analysing what you do like this will not only give you a good idea of how healthy you are but it will allow you to identify some action steps to take moving forwards.

The hot air balloon
When looking at your lifestyle I like to use the analogy of a hot air balloon where the height the balloon is in the sky analogous to your level of health. Think of the chemical, physical and emotional stressors in your life like the sandbags. The more of them you are carrying around the lower you will fly and the greater the risk of crashing down to earth. On the other hand think of the positive steps you can take to improve your chemical, physical and emotional environment as the burner. The more you address these requirements, the more hot air you create and the higher your balloon (health) soars. And of course the higher you soar, the bigger the margin for error you have if someone throws on a couple of extra sandbags. In the same way by taking the action steps to minimise the stressors and maximise your resistance will not only help you achieve a higher level of health and wellness than you ever imagined it will provide a fantastic insurance policy against any unexpected health challenges.

Does that mean we have to start living in caves and revert to a hunter-gatherer lifestyle?
Of course not. Don't get me wrong, I love my mod cons as much as anyone – I am sitting here writing this on my laptop right now. What it means is we need to alter the way we eat, think and move so that our modern lifestyle is more in tune with our bodies'

needs.

What it also means is that you need to take personal responsibility for your health status. Very few people are unhealthy because they have bad genes. In fact if you look at the field of epigenetics, you will find that your lifestyle can have a massive effect on your genetic expression as well. Very few people are unhealthy because of bad luck, and very few people are unwell because of germs that a healthy body wouldn't have been able to handle. Most people are unhealthy because of an unhealthy lifestyle that in incompatible with their body's needs. The thing about this is that it means that no one but you can make you healthy again. You can't rely on a magic pill, because we know that whilst this will cover the symptoms, no one else can do it for you. So if you want to get healthy, it is time to step up. Don't worry because the whole premise of *How To Eat An Elephant* is that I am going to show you exactly how to do it and it is going to be much easier than you think.

But aren't I too old, too sick, too fat, too far gone to get my health back on track?

NO! You are never too old to get healthier. Remember, when I am talking about getting you back to 100 per cent, I am talking about you getting back to your full potential. I can guarantee you no matter how bad (or good) you are right now, there are things you can do to be better and healthier. Of course your full potential may be different to someone else's for a variety of reasons. You may have a genuine genetic disorder, you may have caused some irreversible damage to your body, you may not be as young as you used to be. Whatever it is, it doesn't matter. *How To Eat an Elephant* is going to help you get back closer to YOUR full potential.

How to Eat an Elephant, then, is all about how to create a healthy environment for your body in a way which is congruent with our evolution as hunter gatherers, but still allows us to live in the modern world. The diet is based around real foods. By that I mean foods that grow in nature and do not need to be man-made. So basically fresh fruits and vegetables, nuts and seeds, healthy meats and clean fresh water (as well as fresh air). The exercise is based around the kind of exercise a cave man or woman would have had. It is well-rounded and it is functional. It includes the nine different skills of real fitness as described by the cross-fit principles (strength, power, endurance, flexibility, accuracy, stamina, agility, balance and coordination). All of these our ancestors would have had in spades, and so should we. Finally, *How to Eat an Elephant* is going to teach you how to create a positive mind frame that is going to be congruent with your new lifestyle and is going to help you keep down your stress level and promote a healthy mind and body.

AND it is going to be EASY!

This all sounds a bit extreme. What about everything in moderation?

Did your mum used to say to you to 'do everything in moder-ation'? What does that mean? Should we only love our family in moderation? Should we eat a moderate amount of known carcinogens? Should everyone smoke a moderate amount? Of course not. This saying probably goes back many generations to when there weren't so many unhealthy options. If all you had available to eat was fruit and vegetables, nuts and seeds and good quality meats, then eating a moderate amount of all of them made sense. But the world has changed. There are now many things in your environment, in your cupboards, in your grocery store, in the air and even in your minds that your body doesn't want in any amounts, and by suggesting you do, you are only fooling yourself. Most of the time 'everything in moder-ation' is really only used as a convenient excuse to not change a habit that you know you should change.

One of the biggest problems we face is that our bodies are just so darned good at adapting. So many of these small stressors that we take 'in moderation' don't cause immediate effects. In fact we might not notice any symptoms at all for years or even decades. But eventually these things add up and the cumulative effect of these stressors means that your body is simply not functioning as well as it should be. What makes this even more of a problem is that it happens so gradually – in fact often so slowly that we don't even realise it has happened. Or even worse, we just assume it is 'normal'. For many people this means that they are functioning quite poorly and they don't even know it. Or perhaps they do have symptoms, but they just assume that happens to everyone, or that it is just bad luck.

So forget about doing things 'in moderation'; give your body as near as possible exactly what it needs, and as near as possible none of what it doesn't, and you will find a new, better level of 'normal'.

So what about supplements?

You will notice that all of the solutions in this book revolve around foods rather than supplements and this is done deliberately. I find that too often people use vitamins and minerals as replacements rather than supplements. People assume that they can go on eating a poor diet and that is ok because they are getting the nutrients they need from a pill. This simply isn't the case and for two reasons. Firstly some foods (such as grains and cereals or soy products) can act as what are called anti-nutrients; they can actually interfere with the absorption of nutrients. This means if your diet is not right, you may not be absorbing the goodness from those expensive supplements anyway. Secondly even if you are all getting all the good stuff you need from the pill you are still getting the bad stuff from the poor diet, you are by definition not as healthy as you would be if you changed your diet. So by all means look into vitamins and minerals to supplement the healthy diet you will develop using this book but remember they are a supplement not a replacement.

So how do you eat an elephant?

Well as the saying goes, one bite at a time!

Have you ever wondered why dieting doesn't work? Or why most people let their gym memberships lapse shortly after joining? Or why that positive thinking book or seminar wears off a few weeks after you attended it? The reason is usually that you haven't really committed to change. You have decided to 'give it a go' or you have set yourself a short-term goal. Or you have simply tried to bite off more than you can chew. This often means that what you are trying to change is often simply too hard, or there isn't enough margin for error. Or even worse, you don't really believe you can make the change stick.

If you want to make real change in your life then you need to make a commitment for life. Whatever you decide to change needs to change forever. Sounds hard, doesn't it? But it needn't be. The trick is to eat that elephant one bite at a time. This means small steps of continuous and never-ending health improvement.

So what does this mean for you and your lifestyle changes? Well, the best way to make big changes it to make them slowly, one small step at a time. So pick a small change that is easy for you to make, that you are prepared to make for the rest of your life, and do it. Once you have mastered that one, pick another. If you do this once a month over the course of a year, just imagine how much healthier you will be in 12 months' time!

Health is a journey, not a destination

This book is designed to be a reference book for the rest of your life. You will never be perfect, no one is (and I certainly am not). It doesn't matter if you redo a step 100 times. Your goal is not to be perfect, but to make continuous, never-ending improvement.

How to read this book

Now I don't intend to really tell you how to read this book. You can read it however you like; that's what wellness is about after all, taking charge of your health and making your own informed decisions. But you might like to know how I intended the book to be used. My idea was that you read the index. Pick whichever lifestyle step jumps out to you as being the best and easiest change you can make over the next three weeks and do it. Remember to do it one step at a time. The idea is that you want to make it easy for yourself. If it is fun and easy you will feel good about it and about yourself. You will also notice health changes. This means that when it comes time to pick another step you will be much more enthused and much more likely to succeed. The more success you have, the more change you will make. It is like one big snowball rolling along, gathering momentum.

The last thing you want to do is break that momentum, and this is often where we get it so very wrong. Often we stop the momentum before it has really even started. The easiest way to do this is to try to do something that is too hard, or to try and do too much. This leads to feelings of failure, anger and resentment and blocks you from taking more action in the future. Remember that your goal should be to become as healthy as you can be in five years or 50 years – not to be healthy next week. You have the rest of your life to work on this, so there is no rush.

Why three weeks?

You will notice that a number of the *How To Eat An Elephant* challenges call for three weeks of action. It is said that it takes 21 days to make or break a habit. Remember, this is just to break the habit; not to beat the addiction. I have found with myself and my clients that if you are able to do something successfully for 21 days, you have a really good chance of being able to do it long-term. Twenty-one days is enough time for you to not only break a habit, but also to feel the difference. Once you start to feel different you are much more likely to feel good about the change and keep it going. For the weekly challenges I have found that 3 times really isn't enough for people to create a lifelong habit and I found that 21 weeks was longer than necessary and quite frankly a bit scary for most people. 7 weeks seems to do the trick perfectly.

What if I make the change and don't feel any different?

Many people will get disheartened when they make a massive lifestyle change and don't feel any different. Remember, though, that there are a lot of different factors at play here.

To give an example of this I need to look no further than the Panda's at my local Adelaide Zoo. Adelaide has been abuzz with the arrival of these new animals and with good reason. Not only are they super cute, they are also very rare. There are only several thousand Giant Panda's left in the wild so conservation efforts and breeding programs are very important. There are even less of these beautiful animals in captivity so we need to make sure that the breeding conditions in our zoos are just right. It is no good just feeding them the right stuff. We know that they also need mental stimulation and just the right amount of exercise to ensure that the breeding program is a success. It is easy to see that if we added one of these components without the others it may not make a difference. If we exercised them regularly and kept them mentally stimulated but fed them lollies the chances of success would be slim. Similarly it has been shown that if they are well looked after but kept in a small cage they are very unlikely to breed. If we want to have an effective breeding program we need to make sure they are getting well rounded exercise, are mentally stimulated, are not stressed and are getting the just the right amount and type of bamboo and our bodies are just the same, though thankfully with slightly different nutritional requirements. So remember making one change may not make all the difference, but making many changes certainly will. So start planning to give your body all the nutrients it needs, all the movement it needs, all the positive thoughts it needs, remove any interference and give it a little time, and you WILL start to perform better just like the panda, and you WILL feel the difference.

What if I fail?

When you are alive and creating a lifetime plan, there is no such thing as failing. You are learning and adapting. You will no doubt find that there will be steps you attempt in this book that you will not master in 21 days (or 7 weeks). You will find that there are other steps that you do master only to revert back days, weeks, months or even years later. Do not see this as failure; see it as a learning experience. Start to notice how you feel. Not just how you feel as you are doing the actual action, but how you feel afterwards. If you hoe into a massive chocolate bar for instance, you may feel fantastic whilst you stuff it down, but the next day you are probably going to feel flat and tired and maybe even a little sick. If you keep doing it you will gain weight, lose energy, etc. So judge what you do by the long-term effects. Then, use that knowledge the next time you try that same challenge and it will help you do it better. So long as you are taking on new challenges you are still in the game.

I like to think of this process a little like a rock climber climbing a wall. He knows where he is starting from and he knows where he wants to end up. Ideally he would like to go straight up the wall on the shortest possible path and get there in the least amount of time. Upon starting the journey, though, he finds it is a little tougher than he anticipated. He realises that he needs to detour to the sides at certain stages. In a few spots he even needs to go back a little in order to go forwards. He does not see these detours as failures, though; merely necessary detours on his path to success (the top of the cliff). This is how I would like you to look at these challenges. There is no failure – only necessary detours! When 'failure' happens, you have three choices. You can throw the book in the bin and give up on your journey, you can decide to attempt the same challenge again, or you can select another challenge that you feel is going to be easier for you right now. Remember: the goal of *How to Eat an Elephant* is to make things as easy as possible for yourself.

'But this detour wasn't necessary,' I hear you say. 'I failed!' Well, if you took it, it was necessary. There is obviously still something you need to learn, or else you wouldn't have detoured. Keep at it: the summit is still in sight, and the only thing that can stop you getting there is you.

Can you help me stay on track?

There are two answers to this, yes and no! I cannot really help you stay on track. Only you can do that. However, I can help you help yourself. Picking up this book and re-reading the relevant chapter whenever you are feeling a little weakness (and it will happen) is a great idea. So when you are in the process of conquering a challenge, keep the book handy at all times. Secondly, I have created a website that will help you stay on track. You can log into what challenge you are up to, and it will send you emails reminding you to stay on track and congratulating you on your progress. You get to choose how often you want these emails, so it won't nag you, and if you do happen to fall off the wagon it will help you either restart the same challenge or select a new, easier one.

What if I can't afford to make that change?

There is no doubt that there will be some steps in *How to Eat an Elephant* that will cost money, for example switching to organic food. Remember that a little bit of time and/or money invested in your health now may mean a lot of time and/or money saved later. The best financial investment you can ever make isn't in shares or houses, it is in your health. The returns on investment in terms of savings are better than virtually any other investment you can imagine. For example, consider this: for every dollar spent in Australia on getting people to quit smoking, we save $50. Another study has shown that investing in regular chiropractic care can lead to less x-rays and MRIs, less surgeries and less back pain related costs. In fact even when the cost of the chiropractic care was factored in, these people had lower overall health care expenditures. In other words these people got healthier and saved money at the same time.

The other thing that people often miss is that when you invest time in your health, you actually gain time as well. For every hour that you spend in the gym, you will regain several hours. You will have more energy and enthusiasm and you will be more productive. So much so that the time you gain in increased productivity will be more than the time you invested getting fit. And that is not the only time you will gain.

Did you know that in 2003, males could expect on average to experience 18.6 years of life with a disability, whereas females could expect 20.7 years of life lived with a disability? So despite the fact that we are living longer, there is a large chunk of our lives that we are effectively 'losing'. By investing in our health now we can reduce our chances of the lifestyle diseases that are driving those morbidity stats up. There is no question from the research that by changing our lifestyles we can reduce our risks of strokes, cancers, diabetes and heart attacks. This means that we can not only increase our lifespan but we can increase our productive lifespan as well.

Don't see time and money spent on health as an expense, see it as an investment. Any time and money that you spend on changing the way you think, changing the way you eat or changing the way you move is going to come back to you with interest, often more interest than you realise is possible – and certainly more than you could ever hope to gain by putting your money in the bank.

So start to look at what you are really spending your money on. Often you will find that it doesn't come down to whether you can afford to be healthy, but how highly you prioritise your health. Often I will speak to people who say that they can't afford to get healthy, who spend money on cigarettes, or gambling, or a fancy car or holiday. What they are really saying is that they value those things more than their health. That is OK so long as they realise that is what they are doing.

Having said that, if you have assessed where you are spending your money and evaluated it against your priorities and you still feel that you cannot afford to make that change, then that challenge is simply not the right one for you to do right now. You may feel that it is the one that will have the most significant change for you, but if it is not the easiest, then it must come later. Pick another challenge, perhaps one that will help you save money (like drinking water) and then use that saved money for your health later on.

So where to now?

Now it is time for action. All the talk and good intention in the world will be no good to you at all if you don't take action. So start NOW, don't procrastinate. Know that if you put this book down now without picking a challenge and getting started, the likelihood of you ever doing so is reduced dramatically. Think back to all of those times when you decided that you were going to make a change for the better, when you were going to change when you created a new year's resolution and it never even got off the ground and vow that this time it is going to be different. Remember all I am asking you to do is take one small step, the easiest one you can find in the whole book and do it. Turn the page and get started **NOW!**

The *How to Eat an Elephant* challenges

The following index contains **97** challenges for you to choose from. They are deliberately not sorted into any groups. The reason is that I find often people only focus on diet, or only focus on exercise or think that thinking right is everything. The truth is that you need to look at all of these things if you want to be truly healthy so I have left them jumbled up to ensure you look at all the possibilities and find the best one for you right now.

1. Create a statement of purpose
2. Do functional exercise
3. Drink more water
4. Eat fruit
5. Communicate effectively
6. Eat vegetables
7. Set some goals
8. Snack on healthy stuff
9. Eat eggs
10. Eat less processed carbohydrates
11. Eat less processed sugars
12. Drink less milk
13. Healthy cooking and storing utensils
14. Eat a variety of foods
15. Get a variety of exercise
16. Find a wellness coach
17. Groom yourself healthily
18. Improve your posture
19. Make informed birthing choices
20. Set up your desk
21. Focus on the long term
22. Get more sunlight
23. Remove trans fats

24. Say no to artificial sweeteners
25. Kick pessimism
26. Eat healthy meats
27. Eat organic food
28. Reduce your alcohol consumption
29. Start stretching
30. Get a good bed and pillow
31. Eat a healthy breakfast
32. Minimise antibacterial products
33. Interpret the health info
34. Consume less caffeine
35. Become an inverse paranoid
36. Eat less salt
37. Allocate some 'me time'
38. Eat local
39. Eat more fibre
40. Incorporate some balance exercise
41. Be informed on vaccination
42. Keep your healthy probiotics
43. Check your nervous system
44. Don't fall for marketing spin
45. Allow time for unwinding
46. Be aware of your perception
47. Focus on getting healthy
48. Exercise intensely
49. Get some resistance exercise
50. Do some cardio exercise
51. Minimise medications
52. Use healthy cooking oils
53. Stop smoking
54. Exercise accurately
55. Don't feel guilty
56. Reduce repetitive micro-trauma
57. Start crawling

58. Meditate
59. Breast feed
60. Focus on normal not common
61. Cook at home
62. Do power training
63. Improve your agility
64. Add exercise to your daily routine
65. Get enough movement
66. Use affirmations
67. Utilise mentors and mates
68. Have a healthy scepticism
69. Defeat fear
70. Eat small fish
71. Eat some whole grains
72. Drink healthy juice
73. Healthy eating ratios
74. Don't shop hungry
75. Create a vision board
76. Get a good sleep
77. Focus on what you can control
78. Good time management
79. Grow your own food
80. Make your own baby food
81. Get into nature
82. Invest time
83. Use healthy oils and fats
84. Be informed
85. Find resources
86. Be congruent and honest
87. Maintain your power
88. Minimize chlorine
89. Reduce household toxins
90. Drink bottles and containers
91. Go barefoot

92. Get in control of your money
93. Healthy rewards
94. Maintain your curiosity
95. Running right
96. Eat less un-fermented soy
97. Avoid fluoride

1. Create a statement of purpose

It has been said that most people overestimate what they can do in a day and underestimate what they can do in a lifetime. I find this runs perfectly true for my experience in practice. So often people come in and tell me all of their big plans about how they are going to change their diet, exercise more, start thinking positively and give up smoking... all this week! Whilst I am always supportive and encouraging I also try and help them make their goals more realistic and encourage them to make some longer term goals. On the other hand when it comes to really big long term goals and dreams, far too many people dismiss them as impossibilities because they can't see how they could ever get there.

The truth is you don't need to be able to see how you are going to get there, and you certainly don't need to get there this week! In fact you may never get there, but that doesn't mean it's not a great vision. You see, true health is a journey not a destination, and you have the rest of your life to try and get there. You do need to know where you are trying to get to, though. Without that you are likely to be just walking around in circles regardless of how good your intentions are.

Put simply, you need to figure out all the things you really want in life – be they relationships, family, money, health, fitness, cars, jobs, whatever it is – and create a statement of purpose that reflects them. The point of this exercise is to aim high. Work out what you truly desire and include it. You may not be able to see any way that you can achieve it right now, but you don't need to. The very act of putting it on your mission statement means that you are instructing your mind to look out for these very opportunities. Opportunities that perhaps you may have not noticed, had you not put it in your statement of purpose!

Of course your vision will not be realised without action. So the next step will be to create goals and actions; smaller steps that will help lead you to your bigger vision. But for now, it is time to concentrate on the bigger picture.

There are a few simple rules for a statement of purpose.

1. It should state who you are, what you do, what you stand for and why you do it.
2. It should reflect who you are when you are fulfilling your purpose not necessarily who you are now. (i.e. if you are currently a smoker and drinker but your purpose is to be clean living, then your statement will say clean living).
3. It should be in present tense ('I am' not 'I will be').
4. It should be positive ('I do' not 'I do not').
5. It should be grand. It should get you excited when you read it.
6. It should reflect all facets of your life. Health, wealth, happiness, family, business and relationships.
7. You should not hold anything back based on fear or because it is 'unrealistic'.

The Challenge: In the next 21 days create a personal statement of purpose. Repeat this challenge regularly as you will find over time your purpose will gradually change.

2. Do functional exercise

Have you ever thought about why people really exercise? Some people exercise to feel good, others exercise to look good. Some people exercise so they can say they did, and still more do it for the social aspect. But for me, there is really only one reason to exercise, and that is to stay healthy. By that I mean to make sure my body is in the best possible shape in order to meet the demands of my lifestyle… be that playing cricket, playing with my son, achieving at work or dancing the night away.

So when it comes to my fitness regime, it is really important to me that it is functional. What that means is that the exercise mirrors the challenges I am likely to face in my daily life. I mean, look at a bench press. How often are you really lying flat on your back trying to push a heavy weight up off of your chest? Or what about running a marathon – how often are you going to need to run for four hours on end to get through your day?

There are some activities, though, that you are likely to need to do all of the time. Every time I pick up my son I need to do a squat. Every time I get up from lying down I do a sit-up, and when I field in cricket I do sprints and jumps. This sort of exercise not only trains the right muscles (including the ones you don't see) but if you are doing it right, it also teaches them to work in unison in order to get the job done in a safe efficient way. Bear in mind when doing functional exercise, though, form is every-thing. Rather than training until you can't go any more, train until you can't do it with the correct technique any more.

You will also find that this kind of exercise will allow you to do a more intense workout in a shorter period of time. It will also ensure that your body is not only better at doing your daily activ-ities but also less likely to get injured whilst doing so. So get into functional fitness and get your body ready for life!

The challenge: Start making your exercise more functional. One session a week for 7 weeks start incorporating more complex activities (like squats or lunges) and fewer machines. Repeat as many times as it takes until all your exercise is functional.

3. Drink more water

A News poll survey conducted by BRITA Water Filter Systems found that Australians are chronically dehydrated with 4.5 million adults (30per cent of the population) only drinking three glasses or less of water each day, well under the recommended minimum daily intake of eight to ten glasses.

For the first time last year water was formally recognised as an 'essential nutrient' in the revised National Health & Medical Research Council (NHMRC) Nutrient Reference Values for Australia and New Zealand.

The guidelines recommend that Australians need to increase their absolute minimum intake to eight to 10 glasses to prevent dehydration. For optimal performance however this value can be increased again. A good guide if you want to perform at your best is to drink 25-25mls of water for every kg of body weight. So for a 60kg female that would be around 1.5-2L whilst for a 85-90kg male it would be around 2-3L. If you exercise a lot, the weather is hot, you're pregnant or you drink lots of diuretics (tea, coffee, alcohol, soft drinks), then drink even more.

Remember also that these totals are for water only. You should not include any other drinks in this. In fact many of the other things we drink are diuretics and actually serve to leach water out of our systems. Non-caffeinated herbal teas can be a nice warming substitute for the tea and coffee when the temperature drops.

If you do decide to make some changes to your beverage intake remember that you don't need to do it all at once. In fact it is actually better for you to make these changes gradually. Slowly increase your intake of water and reduce your intake of tea (caffeinated), coffee, alcohol and soft drinks and enjoy the changes in your health and your performance.

The Challenge: Drink one extra glass of water each day for the next 21 days. Attempt this challenge as many times as you need until you are drinking 1L of water each day for every 25kg you weigh.

4. Eat fruit

There are so many good reasons to eat more fruit that I don't even know where to start. And you probably don't need me to either. We all know that eating fruit is good for us. But just for arguments sake let's look at the benefits in terms of cancer alone.

For many people a cancer scare can be an opportunity to reassess their lives, to really analyse what they have being doing with their health and how they have ended up in the situation they are in – be it the way that they eat, exercise or think – or all of the above.

Here are some compelling studies showing the link between what you eat and your risk of cancer.

- Consumption of fruits and vegetables is associated with a lowered risk of lung cancer, skin cancer and colon cancer.
- People who eat the most apples are 58per cent less likely to get lung cancer than those who eat the least.
- Men who consume most of their fibre from vegetables are 18per cent less likely to develop prostate cancer.
- Sugar intake is a strong risk factor that contributes to higher breast cancer rates, particularly in older women.
- Men whose average intake of lycopene (an antioxidant abundant in tomatoes) is 19 milligrams each day have a 16per cent lower risk of prostate cancer than men who take three milligrams.
- Broccoli and tomatoes, both of which have been previously found to help fight cancer, have been found to be even more effective against prostate cancer when eaten together as part of a daily diet.
- Fish oil consumption can delay or reduce tumour development in breast cancer.
- High carotene intake (found in carrots) – especially high alpha-carotene intake – significantly reduces the risk of

ovarian cancer.

- Men who eat small amounts of onions, garlic, scallions, shallots and leeks each day decrease their risk of prostate cancer by more than 33per cent.
- Prostate cancer risk was significantly higher in a group of men with the lowest selenium (found in brazil nuts and walnuts) blood levels.
- Prostate cancer patients who added three tablespoons of ground flaxseed daily to their diet had more slowly-dividing tumour cells and a greater rate of tumour cell death.
- Women with the highest intakes of folate (found in leafy green vegetables) were 40per cent less likely to develop cancer of the colon and rectum.
- Individuals in the top 20per cent in terms of weekly fruit and vegetable consumption had a 25per cent lower risk of developing stomach cancer than those in the bottom 20per cent.

I have included all of these studies here in the hope that you will not be one of those people who waits until they have a massive scare before they decide to reassess their lives. If you want to create health in your life and reduce your risk of chronic disease later in life, the time to start is now. Early detection is good. Prevention is better than early detection. Wellness is even better again, ensuring that you are not just avoiding getting sick but your body is in fact functioning to its full potential. Of course the reason to eat a healthy diet is not just to avoid cancer. Your goal should be to get healthy. If you eat the foods that your body is designed to eat you naturally decrease your cancer risk, find your ideal weight and improve your immune system function.

The Challenge: Eat one extra piece of fresh fruit each day for the next 21 days. Attempt this challenge as many times as you need to get to 2-3 pieces of fresh fruit daily.

5. Communicate effectively

Anthony Robbins says that "the quality of your life is determined by the quality of your communication", and whilst this might be overstating the case a little bit it certainly suggests just how important communication is for your life and for your health. 'But how can communication affect my health?' I hear you ask. Well, it's all about stress. In particular, the unnecessary stress that goes hand-in-hand with poor communication.

How many times have you been having a huge argument with someone, or experiencing trouble sealing a deal at work, or find yourself in trouble with your better half – and when it all comes down to it you realise that you were really arguing about nothing. In fact either you both actually agreed, or there was in fact a readily agreeable compromise that was easy to find once you both started opening your ears rather than your mouths. And really, at the end of the day, that sentence holds the key.

Asking great questions and listening really is the key to great communication. So often we think that the key to communication is being able to get our points of view across as well as we can. However that is not communicating, that is just talking. The key to communication is not about winning but being able to see the other person's point of view in order to find a mutually agreeable solution moving forward. This enables you to create effective long-term partnerships with people and sets up mutually beneficial relationships that not only mean less stress now but also less stress in the future. So next time you are in a conversation that is not going so well, try asking 'What can I do here to help us create a solution to this problem?'

And don't forget that it is not just about the communication between yourself and others – the way you communicate with yourself may be even more important. Lots of people talk to themselves in a way that they would never allow others to do.

Lies, put-downs, fear mongering and focusing on problems rather than solutions can form part of this internal communication all too often. So when it comes to self-talk (and we all do it), try to use the same rules. Try to figure out what it is that you really want and focus on finding solutions that will help get you there. This self-talk affects our health in so many ways. So often it stop us from finding emotional peace and happiness, it stops us from taking action on our health and it allows us to eat, think and move in ways that are just not healthy.

The good news is that the more you consciously create this positive self-talk, the more the negative will fade away.

The challenge: For the next 21 days focus on communicating rather than talking and focus on solutions that work well for everyone.

6. Eat vegetables

Ok this one should really go without saying but having a look around at most people's diets it seems like there are plenty of people who didn't listen to their mum. Vegetables really are the number one thing you can eat for your health. But don't fall into the trap of thinking that one 'super' vegetable is going to save you, there is no such thing. Sure there are plenty of vegetables that are great for you and have fantastic health benefits but no vegetable is all things to all people. You need a good variety of as many different vegetables as possible to make sure that you get all the nutrients you need.

So why are vegetables so darned good?

Well they are chock full of vitamins including A, B, C and K and minerals and they are the best source of dietary fibre. They are also full of anti-oxidants, in fact what many people don't realise when they reach for the latest marketed, hyped anti-oxidant super food that you can get all the antioxidants you ever need from your veggies.

As a result vegetable intake has been linked to decreased risk of heart disease, cancers, strokes and diabetes as well as much more. In fact research from the International Journal of cancer has shown that men can lower their risk of prostate cancer by simply eating their veggies. Men who consumed most of their fibre from vegetables were 18 per cent less likely to develop prostate cancer, whereas those who received their fibre from fruits or grains didn't show a decrease in prostate cancer risks.

Don't forget that the more you cook your vegetables the more nutrients they lose. So don't boil them til they are a pale yellow like Grandma used to. A light steam is the best way to cook them and still retain their value.

So although you already know you should eat your veggies now it is time to act. Eat a broad range of vegetables (the less

34

cooked the better) with every meal. Your body will thank you for it and you will feel great.

The challenge: Eat one extra vegetable each day for the next 21 days that is different to the vegetables you currently eat. Attempt this challenge as many times as you like until you eat 8-9 serves of vegetables a day.

7. Set some goals

Goal-setting is all about creating action. It is about taking your grandest visions and your wildest dreams (be they health, wealth, happiness or love) and taking a step in the right direction. Note that I said just a step, because goal-setting is also about not getting too far ahead of yourself.

Of course there is no point taking a step until you know where you are going. So before you start setting yourself goals, you had better have a grand vision in place, otherwise you are just going to be meandering around in circles like a sheep in a paddock. So first you need to create a mission statement (chapter 1) and perhaps a vision board (chapter 76) and work out what it is that you truly desire in life.

Once you have that big idea, then you are ready to start creating goals. When I think of goal-setting I always think of the rock climber I mentioned in the intro. She knows she wants to get the top (the vision/mission) but until she has done it, she has no idea how she is going to get there. What she can work out, though, is what her next step needs to be: she needs to reach her hand up and grab onto that next ledge.

So when you are creating goals, try and find out what the next step is in moving you towards your mission. What can you do right now, this week or even this year that is going to get you closer to where you want to be? Ensure that whatever the goal is it is measurable and achievable. Once you work out what that goal is, write it down somewhere where you will look at it constantly – where it will always be fresh in your mind – and then start taking action! After all, there is no point having a goal if you never act on it.

Now it may be that in the course of her ascent, the rock climber needs to go sideways, or diagonally, or even at times back down a little, but she always maintains her mission: to get to the top. It is OK to change your goal or even to cast it aside altogether if you realise that it isn't getting you where you want to be. Or perhaps you have embarked on an entirely new mission. Just replace it with a newer, better goal and continue on the journey. So long as you keep setting goals and keep focussing on your mission, the only thing that can stop you from getting there is you.

In fact this book is entirely designed around this idea of goal setting and how to make it easy for you. Each challenge is in essence a goal, so if you want to start real easy just use one of these challenges as your first goal. No doubt in time, though, you will have other goals that exist outside of the pages of this book as well.

The challenge: In the next 21 days set yourself a goal. Make it measurable and achievable and write it down somewhere you will see it. Repeat this challenge at regular intervals for the rest of your life.

8. Snack on healthy stuff

Remember when mum used to say "stop snacking, you'll ruin your dinner"? Well, now you can go back and tell your mum that the latest research shows that consuming small portions of healthy foods throughout the day is in fact the best way to eat.

Research shows many health benefits from eating repeated small snacks including weight loss, improved glucose tolerance, reduced appetite (by 27per cent), reduced cholesterol levels (9per cent), reduced insulin levels (28per cent) and reduced cortisol levels (17per cent). This means that by snacking healthily, you will have a reduced chance of strokes, heart disease and diabetes, some of the biggest killers going around.

Eating lots of smaller snacks also helps your body feel full and maintain a more consistent energy level for a longer period of time. This is because small amounts of slow-burning food release a more consistent flow of glucose sugars into your bloodstream, rather than a sudden spike in sugar insulin followed by a 'crash and burn' (followed by a craving for more sugary foods).

The most important thing about snacking is to choose healthy foods. You want to eat things that maintain your energy levels for long periods of time, so that the sugars are absorbed into your bloodstream more slowly. But remember, even if a food is low G.I. (slow burning), it's not always necessarily healthy. For example, ice cream is low G.I., but it is obviously better to choose something like nuts and seeds, wholegrains (limited amounts), vegetables (preferably raw), fruit (limited amounts, due to their high carb content), or cold meats (cold, not processed). Also remember that sugary drinks (i.e. soft drinks or fruit juices) will cause the same spikes and troughs in energy levels as sugary snacks.

Also remember that peanuts are legumes not nuts and are not the healthiest snacks to have. They have a high Omega 6 to

Omega 3 fat ratio (which is bad) and they are also prone to a carcinogenic mould called aflatoxin. This means that you are either at risk of this carcinogenic mould or there will be incredibly high levels of pesticides to ensure it is killed off. I know it is annoying that I am recommending you avoid the most readily-available, cheapest 'nuts' on the market, but it is what it is. By all means eat plenty of real nuts (assuming no allergy), cashews, walnuts, brazil nuts and almonds. They are a great source of protein, healthy fats, fibre and many vitamins.

Plan your healthy snacks for the week when grocery shopping and put them on your desk or close at hand, so if you do feel like a snack during the day, that's the first thing you'll reach for.

The challenge: Change your snacks one day a week for the next 7 weeks to include only healthy nuts, healthy meats, fruits, vegetables and water with a good mix of each especially those snacks that are high in protein. Attempt this challenge as many times as it takes until you are doing it 7 days a week.

9. Eat eggs

Many people, especially those on a diet or watching their cholesterol, try to steer clear of eggs. However research from the *American Journal of Clinical Nutrition* has now shown that eating two eggs a day helps to maintain LDL/HDL cholesterol levels, and numerous other studies have shown that eggs do not increase your risk of heart disease.

In fact eggs are a fantastic source of protein that can help to balance out your diet. Most of our Western diets contain way too many carbohydrates and sugars and nowhere near enough protein. As well as protein, eggs also contain essential amino acids, vitamins and even anti-oxidants that help prevent macular degeneration and eye disorders.

Of course there are eggs and there are eggs, so what makes a healthy egg?

Organic- Obviously the fewer chemicals involved in the process the better. Not only will you not have to ingest those toxins, the egg will be healthier too.

Free range- Obviously a free range chicken is going to be healthier. It has more space, more muscle, less disease and stronger bones. This means healthier eggs.

Grass fed- If possible, grass fed eggs are the best but not always easy to find. They have much healthier fat profiles than those from chickens fed purely on grains. You may need to find a friend with a farm or keep your own chooks to make sure they are grass fed.

Raw- Now you may not want to eat all your eggs raw, but raw eggs have higher amounts of healthy anti-oxidants than cooked ones. Check out my breakfast juice for an easy, tasty way to get some raw eggs into your diet. Remember, your risk of getting salmonella from healthy raw eggs is incredibly low.

So eat your eggs and your body will thank you for it. Up to

two a day has been shown to be very good for you.

The challenge: Eat one extra egg based meal each week for the next 7 weeks. Attempt this challenge as many times as it takes until you are eating at least 3 eggs a week (and up to 14).

10. Eat less processed carbohydrates

Is it time to revise the food pyramid?

Over millions of years humans have evolved to eat a diet of primarily wild animals and vegetation and our genes have changed very little in the last 100,000 years. Yet in the last few thousand years our diets (and our lives) have changed remarkably.

In fact it is estimated that the first grain was harvested and domesticated in South West Asia around 9,000 years ago and even then it would have been a much smaller part of the diet than it is today. As a result we have not had time to evolve to process our modern diets, in particular the high consumption of processed grains and sugars. Any meal or snack high in grains or refined sugar generates a rapid rise in blood glucose. When there is more sugar than your body requires for its current needs it is stored for the future. Your pancreas secretes insulin to store the sugar for future requirements. Some sugar is stored in the liver and muscles but not as much as most people think. In fact the amount of sugar stored in muscles and the liver is not even enough for one active day. Anything over and above that is stored as fat. This is your body saving for rainy day (a drought or famine). In our modern society and with our western diets, these famines never come. We always have more sugar and carbohydrates than we need available to us.

Any sudden increase in blood sugar from grains or refined sugars leads to increased insulin. This then rapidly removes the sugar from the blood stream, leading to lowered blood sugar. If ignored long enough, this will lead to a "crash" as a result of hypoglycaemia and low blood sugars.

If these eating habits are maintained over time, the cells will try to protect themselves from the toxic effects of high insulin and hence their receptors become resistant. This means that the

pancreas has to secrete more insulin to get the sam
has to "yell louder" to get the cells to listen. This
vicious cycle, with more resistance leading to
leading to more resistance and so on.

Insulin also has many other effects in the body. High insulin
levels lower your levels of glucagon and growth hormone, both
of which help to burn fat and sugar. It causes hunger (especially
for sweets), leads to decreased vitamin C absorption (lower
immunity), decreased magnesium in muscles (muscle cramps
and constricted blood vessels), increased blood pressure and
heart rate, altered growth hormone levels (decreased bone
formation – osteoporosis), decreased thyroid function and
increased cell division (ageing).

Of course our body needs carbohydrates. They are an
essential part of our diet. The trick is to eat carbohydrates that
are released more slowly and so don't lead to the same sugar
spikes and crashes. The best way to get these "good" carbs is of
course fruit and vegetables, in particular vegetables. And the
best way for them to be eaten is whole and as raw as possible.
This means that all of the fibre and body of the fruit and
vegetables stays intact, ensuring that the carbohydrates are
released slowly and evenly into your body. Not to mention all
the other goodness you get from the fruits and vegetables.

So get your carbohydrates from fruit and vegetables (and
limited whole grains), and you will improve your health and
vitality in more ways than one.

The challenge: Cut out one of your sources of processed
carbohydrates (e.g. bread or cereal or pasta or cakes and
snacks) from your diet for the next 21 days. Attempt this
challenge as many times as it takes until you have eliminated processed grains and cereals completely.

11. Eat less processed sugars

Are you a sweet tooth?

OK, so by now we all know that we have way too much sugar in the average modern diet. It is added to most of our foods in enormous quantities, and if that isn't enough, we often add more – whether in our tea and coffee, smothered over our breakfast and even added to our salad dressings. And if it isn't processed sugars, it is often high fructose corn syrups (read some labels –you will be amazed how much stuff this is added to).

We also know that these sugars increase our blood sugar levels, increase our insulin resistance (diabetes and pre-diabetes), promote weight gain and cause sugar crashes. This in turn can lead to decreased metabolism, increased hunger, lowered immunity, muscle cramps, increased blood pressure and heart disease, osteoporosis, and increased ageing.

So if you haven't done so already, it is time to start decreasing the amount of processed sugars in your diet. The good news is you don't need to go cold turkey. A good way to start is by replacing these processed, refined sugars with more natural sugars. Being more complex molecules, these sugars don't cause such instantaneous rises in blood sugar and hence don't have such drastic effects.

Foods like honey, fruit, maple syrup, molasses and fruit and vegetable juices can be used to provide sweetness to your food in a healthier way. Of course these sweeteners are still really high in carbohydrates so you won't want to overdo it. In fact over time you can begin to reduce your intake of the honey, maple syrup and molasses as well, and start to get most of your sweetness and carbohydrates from fruits and vegetables. But that will take time.

So start reducing your reliance on refined processed sugars. Like any addiction, it may be tough at first but it will be well worth the effort and once you get the hang of it you won't miss the daily sugar crashes.

The challenge: Remove one of your sources of processed sugars from your diet for the next 21 days. Attempt this challenge as many times as it takes until you have removed these sugars from your diet completely.

12. Drink less milk

Are we designed to drink milk?

Are human beings really the only the animal on the planet that requires the milk designed for another species' baby in order to be healthy?

We know that genetically we have changed very little in the last 100,000 years. We also know that it is only in the last 9,000 years or so that we have domesticated cattle and started drinking their milk. So we know that we have not evolved to drink milk, but is it good for us?

According to Eileen Kennedy of the US Department of Agriculture, "There's nothing against vegetable sources of calcium, but we have to fashion healthful eating around current habits." In other words we can get all the calcium we need from vegetables, but it is easier to get people to drink milk than to eat vegetables.

Although milk's calcium and other nutrients do promote bone growth, confirms Dr. T. Colin Campbell, PhD, nutritional biochemist at Cornell University, other substances in dairy foods (certain proteins and especially sodium) actually leach some calcium from bone.

Perhaps this explains why a 12 year Harvard Nurses' Health Study involving 78,000 nurses found that those who drank the most milk – two or more glasses per day – had a slightly higher risk of arm fracture (5 per cent increase) and significantly higher risk of hip fracture (45per centper cent increase).

It may also explain the disparities between calcium intake and bone health that can be seen worldwide. People in countries that consume the highest levels of dairy foods (North American and northern European nations) take in two or three times more calcium, yet break two or three times more bones than people with the lowest calcium intake (Asians and Africans).

Epidemiological research suggests a correlation between milk consumption and at least two kinds of cancer prevalent in Europe and North America: breast and prostate.

In the US Physician's Health Study, researchers tracked 20,885 male doctors over 10 years. Those who consumed at least two and a half servings of dairy food per day were 30 per cent more likely to develop prostate cancer than doctors who consumed less than half a serving.

The challenge: Remove one of your sources of milk (i.e. your cereal, your tea/coffee or your iced coffee) from your diet for the next 21 days. Attempt this challenge as many times as it takes until you have completely removed milk products from your diet.

13. Healthy cooking and storing utensils

We often spend lots of time thinking about the health benefits of what we are going to cook but how often do you think about what you are cooking with?

Non-stick pans are so handy to cook with, especially if you cook like me. No matter how badly you burn it to the pan, it just slides right off. But what is Teflon anyway? And is it really safe to cook with?

Well, non-stick fry pans have been shown to release toxins. In fact Teflon is known to give off a cocktail of 15 types of toxic particles and gases. These chemicals include two carcinogens and a chemical which is deadly to humans at low doses and can be released even under common cooking conditions. In fact there is a condition known as 'teflon flu' that includes headaches, chills, backache and fever.

Add to this the fact that Teflon is produced using a chemical called PFOA which has been linked with cancer, liver damage, growth defects, immune system damage and even death in lab animals and has been ordered to be removed by 2015 by the EPA, and the picture is not looking rosy.

What about aluminium? Aluminium cookware is known to leach the metal into your food and given what we now know about the links between aluminium and Alzheimer's disease, this one may be best to avoid too.

Stainless steel is quite stable, however you need to remember that stainless steel cookware contains alloys of nickel, chromium, molybdenum, carbon, and various other metals. These metals can leech into your food, especially as your cookware gets older.

So what options are left? Well as it turns out, the best options are the most tried and true. Old fashioned glass and ceramic cookware are made of inert materials that have stood the test of time and also withstand the latest research too. So perhaps it is time to pull out mum's old ceramic pots for tonight's dinner!

The challenge: In the next 21 days purchase a piece of glass or ceramic cookware. Repeat this challenge as many times as it takes until you have replaced all of your cookware with glass or ceramics.

14. Eat a variety of foods

Eating the right amounts and the right variety of foods can be just as important as eating the right kinds of food. A good variety of healthy foods is essential to ensure that you get all of the nutrients your body needs because they all have something to offer.

Of course when I talk about variety of foods I don't mean a little McDonalds, a little KFC and a little Pizza Hut, I mean a good variety of healthy foods: fruits and vegetables, nuts and seeds, fish, grass fed meats and water. Nothing more, nothing less.

But even when you are only eating real foods like our ancestors ate, it is still important to consume variety. So if you want to get all of the nutrients your body needs, eat some fish, some grass fed meats (red and white), some seeds and nuts (not peanuts), plenty of water and a good variety of fruits and vegetables. Remember that you should eat more serves of vegetables than you do fruits, and you should eat more of both of these than you do meats.

A good trick for ensuring you eat a good variety of fruits and vegetables is to make sure you have a good assortment of colours. Lots of Aussies load up on carrots and potatoes without eating as many leafy green vegetables, capsicums, eggplants or sweet corn.

So add some variety to your menu – it will not only be better for you but you will add some variety and flavour to your cooking as well.

The challenge: In the next 21 days add 5 new recipes to your repertoire that include only healthy ingredients and a variety of different vegetables. Repeat this challenge as many times as it takes until you are eating a good variety of healthy foods and recipes.

15. Get a variety of exercise

I am constantly having people come in to see me in my practice saying, 'I am fit, I am on my feet all day, I run every day or I go to the gym everyday – aren't I fit?' What these people often don't realise is that there are 9 different aspects to fitness and that you cannot be truly considered fit unless you are able to perform in each of these areas.

The 9 recognised general fitness skills are endurance, stamina, strength, flexibility, power, coordination, agility, balance, and accuracy are spelled out in the Cross-Fit Journal. By definition, if you are not great at any of these 9 facets then your body is performing at less than its best. When your body is not performing at its best, it of course affects your ability to do these physical activities wherever they may crop up in your life. But perhaps more importantly, it affects your overall health.

For instance, it is well known that endurance exercise is good for your heart, but did you know that doing interval training – where your heart rate goes rapidly up, and then recovers – helps to prepare your heart to cope with sudden increases in demand (like when you're stressed), hence reducing your risk of heart attack? Interval training has also been shown to increase metabolic rate, improve lung function and reduce stress.

So as you can see, these 9 different facets of fitness are not just good for your body – they are essential for your body, just like your dietary requirements. They will help you in many more ways than just merely athletic performance.

How can you train in order to exercise all of these 9 areas? The first and most important component is that you need to keep your training regime broad and constantly varied.

Secondly, you need to make sure that you are doing lots of compound activities. If you try and do all 9 components separately, you will be training all day and you still won't get the same effect that you would by doing several together. For example, doing a series of squats correctly can help you to improve your endurance, stamina, strength, flexibility, power, coordination, agility, balance, and accuracy all at once.

To do a complete work-out (using all 9 components and compound activities) will require good technique and will need to be personalised to your level of fitness. So unless you are already very knowledgeable about health and fitness and a wide range of exercises, it may be a good idea to get yourself a personal trainer.

Whatever you do, if you can incorporate some more well-rounded exercise into your regular training routine, you will not only perform better but you will be a lot healthier as well.

The challenge: For the next 21 days add one extra fitness skill to your exercise routine. Attempt this challenge as many times as it takes until you have a well rounded fitness regime.

16. Find a wellness coach

In previous columns I have talked about wellness. Here is a guide to finding a wellness practitioner that best suits you.

Recommendation. Your health and wellness is a very important thing. It would be unwise to choose a practitioner because they are the closest or the cheapest. The best way to find a wellness doctor would be to get a recommendation from a friend, relative or local health food shop that shares your goals for health.

Humility. Your wellness doctor should provide inspiration and advice to empower you to take charge of your health, because ultimately it is your body that does the healing. They should also be a good listener, after all no-one knows more about your body than you do.

Do you "click"? It is a hard thing to define, but if you are going to find a wellness doctor that is going to help you get and stay well for the rest of your life, it is important that you connect with them. You should feel comfortable enough to ask all of the tough questions that you need to ask to discover your true health.

Does the doctor look healthy? The best person to guide you towards health and wellness is someone who has been there and done that. They know the road that you need to take and perhaps made some of the mistakes for you along the way.

Physical, chemical and emotional? Is this person looking at all aspects of health and wellness and are they looking at the body as a whole? All of the cells in your body need to be functioning at their best in order for you to be well. Your wellness doctor needs to understand this and needs to look at the body as a whole rather than just some parts or chemicals in isolation.

How are you being evaluated? Is your doctor assessing you based on how you are feeling or how you are functioning? True wellness means ensuring that your body is functioning as well as it can be at all times – not waiting for symptoms to tell you that something is seriously wrong.

What types of techniques are used? Is the doctor using techniques and advice that you are comfortable with? Are the techniques designed to improve your function and wellness or merely dull the symptoms you are experiencing? Are they proven and safe?

Qualifications? Whatever approach you choose, be sure that they are adequately qualified in that area. They should also have sufficient training to advise you chemically, physically and emotionally - or be prepared to refer you to someone who does.

How much does it cost? You should be informed of the fees and charges up front and in an open and honest way. Be sure that the fees for the care required are within what you are prepared to pay for your health.

Are you are seriously ill or suffering from an acute episode? If so then maybe what you require is more than wellness care - maybe you also need some crisis care to get you through this situation. This may or may not require a different practitioner. But you will also want someone to help you address the underlying causes and help you improve your function in the long run.

Perhaps the wellness profession that best encompasses all of these criteria is chiropractic. Chiropractic is one of the few professions with a five year Masters level degree (chiropractic education has more hours of anatomy, physiology and neurology than a medical degree) that still maintains a wellness philosophy that is holistic and uses functional evaluation and techniques.

The Challenge: Find a health care professional that suits your philosophy and will help you achieve your wellness goals. Attempt this challenge as many times as it takes until you find the right person or people for your needs.

17. Groom yourself healthily

Do you really know what you are putting on your skin, spraying on your body or brushing on your teeth?

Everything you apply to your skin, scalp or other body parts is absorbed by the body's bloodstream. So what exactly are you 'consuming'? Many products are jumping on the wellbeing bandwagon by labeling themselves 'organic', but a product needs to be Certified Organic and contain no artificial preservatives, parabens etc. to be truly good for you. If a product is genuinely natural, it will have a short shelf-life and you should be able to eat it!

More than a third of personal care products contain ingredients linked to cancer. The aluminium in deodorant may be linked to breast cancer, according to a UK study, so try an aluminium-free alternative or 'body crystal'. Check the packaging of your creams, sunscreens and cleansers – if they contain methyl paraben, ethyl paraben, propyl paraben, butyl paraben, isobutyl paraben or E216, look for more natural alternatives. And avoid sodium lauryl sulphate in your shaving creams, soaps, shampoos and body washes – it contains 1,4-dioxane, which is suspected of causing damage to the central nervous system, liver and kidneys. As for cosmetics, try those made from rock minerals which are devoid of nasty fillers such as talc, alcohol, dyes, mineral oil and petroleum, and won't irritate the skin.

There are many natural substances and plant extracts that humans have used for millions of years, such as chamomile for shiny hair and oats for exfoliating dead skin cells. Cleopatra bathed in milk, and the Ancient Greeks rubbed their hair and bodies with olive oil. Our bodies work synergistically with many of these basic substances, so why complicate things by introducing products concocted in laboratories with synthetic ingredients and fragranced with aroma chemicals?

Many of the beauty products that are advertised on television, or which are filling your bathroom shelves right now, have only been on the market for a very short time. Of the nearly four million synthetic chemicals in your environment, less than one per cent of these are known well enough to be able to ascertain their safety. And while some of the products you use every day to shave, wash, moisturise, deodorise and clean your teeth may not be carcinogenic by themselves, the more you combine and layer them, who knows what affects they could be having?

Despite what the big beauty companies tell you, there are no magical shortcuts to beauty! Rather than focusing on a myriad of products and superficial beauty, it's a good diet, exercise and sleep that's going to help you look younger for longer. Remember: the most attractive look is always someone who glows with natural health.

The challenge: Start reading the labels of your personal grooming products and in the next 21 days, replace one that has unhealthy ingredients with a more appropriate one. Repeat this as many times as it takes until you have replaced all of your personal grooming products with healthy ones that you like.

18. Improve your posture

Many people in Australia spend over half of their day in a chair
– be it at work, in the car or driving – and a large portion of them
are not sitting in a suitable posture. This helps to explain why a
study of 88 healthy 20-50 year olds showed that 66 per centper
cent had forward head posture and 38 per cent per centhad an
increased curvature in their mid spines.

How well you maintain your posture can be very important,
and not just for looks. In fact one study has shown that as you get
older your posture becomes particularly important. Looking at
the thoracic kyphosis in elderly people (the amount that your
spine bends forwards between your shoulder blades), it was
shown that a mild increase in the curvature lead to a mortality
rate that was 1.44 times that of the control group whilst a
moderate increase in that curve leads to 2.4 times the mortality
rate. In other words, your risk of dying is related to the degree of
excessive curvature in your spine.

So why does your posture have such a big impact on your
health?

Think of your body like a car. If your car's wheels aren't
aligned properly, your car won't perform as well as it should. It
will suffer from wear and tear and will be more likely to break
down. Your body is exactly the same. For every inch that your
head comes forward there will be up to an extra 15kg of weight
on the muscles at the back of your neck, that's a lot of extra hard
work.

Poor posture can also have a number of other effects on your
body. It can lead to a reduced lung capacity, vascular problems,
digestive problems, increases discomfort and pain, loss of proper
spinal movement, and last but by no means least, interference to
the nervous system that controls and regulates your whole body.

So what does normal posture look like?

From front on, your spine should be nice and straight. This means that your ears should be at the same height, your shoulders should be at the same height and your hips should be at the same height. Many people just assume that this is the case and get a rude shock when they actually look in the mirror. Check it out for yourself, or even better get a friend to check it for you. While you're at it, check out your posture from side on as well. The middle of your ear should be directly above the middle of your shoulder, which should be directly above your hip, which should be above the ball of your ankles.

Ok, so my posture could be better. What can I do about it?

Well, there are a number of things that you need to consider in order to improve your posture.

Firstly, what are the stressors that are causing your posture to be distorted in the first place? Are you sitting in a poor posture at work? Are you doing repetitive, one-sided activities that are causing stress on your spine? Are you anxious, causing excessive tension between your shoulder blades? Try and figure out what your stressors are and reduce them wherever possible.

Next you will need to look at what your body requires in order to maintain proper posture. The most important thing it needs is proper movement and proper stability. When it comes to exercise, it is not just the amount of movement that is important, but the quality of movement. If you are being restricted due to pain or lack of mobility in your spine, then it might be time to get a spinal check up from your health care practitioner.

So make sure that you look after your posture and your spine – it is the only one you have got!

The challenge: Assess your posture or get someone to assess it for you. If you think yours may not be ideal then book an appointment with a chiropractor to get it thoroughly checked.

19. Make informed birthing choices

If you've recently discovered you're pregnant, congratulations! It will bring great joy and great responsibility. You are now in charge of you and your family's health and it would seem responsible to find out everything you can about the choices that will confront you over the next year or so in order to make informed healthy choices, so hopefully this will help.

At hospital or at home?

For many people, this isn't even a choice they consider. They have been brought up through experience, school, TV and society in general to assume that all births happen in a hospital and by a doctor. If you are in a high risk group, this may well be the best option for you, however if you are in the vast majority of people who don't fit that bill then research suggests that a home birth is at least as safe. In fact one large study published by the British *Journal of Medicine* in 2005 showed home births for low-risk pregnancies were as safe as hospital births and had much lower rates of intervention.

If you consider birth to be a healthy, natural process rather than a medical event that needs to be managed, you may wish to birth your baby at home with a private, experienced midwife. If anything unexpected goes wrong, she will be able to advise on what to do, and arrange for you to move to hospital if necessary.

Ultrasounds and tests?

Did you know that the World Health Organisation recommends *against* the routine use of ultrasounds during pregnancy? Why is that? Well, the answer is that as with all interventions, ultra-sounds carry some risks. Research has shown the possibility that ultrasound can cause slowed growth of the fetus and that some children exposed to ultrasound may later have mild neurological deficits. There is also the risk of a false result which may lead to more risky interventions or even termination of the pregnancy. But isn't *not* having an ultrasound risky? Well, one large study in the US of more than 15,000 pregnant women showed no improvement in the mortality rate of the babies undergoing routine ultrasound.

Birth position?

Birth position is a really important choice. If a woman lies flat on her back, her pelvis is tucked in and her birthing canal points towards the ceiling, reducing her pelvic outlet by as much as 30 per cent. She needs to work against gravity, meaning there is more resistance and she is more likely to need some sort of intervention. Squatting may be a more logical choice.

Birthing interventions?

Medical interventions all have risks. Even a routine, scheduled caesarean section with no complication carries twice the risk of mortality for mum. There is also a 20 per cent chance she will get an infection as a result of the surgery which often also leads to antibiotics. More babies born after caesarean section also develop respiratory distress syndrome compared with natural vaginal deliveries.

Twenty-three per cent, or nearly one in four women who are given an epidural will develop a complication, including higher mortality rates, neurological damage and fever. They are also likely to have a longer labour. There is also four times greater use of forceps or vacuum extraction and at least twice the rate of caesarean section after an epidural, which can also be very stressful for the baby, potentially leading to interference to its fragile spine and nervous system. Research also shows that having an epidural also leads to an increased risk of back pain after the event and even one year later.

A healthy, natural birth provides a number of benefits for the baby, including beneficial bacteria that help set up the baby's immune system for life. So if you are expecting, be sure to examine the pro's and con's and make sure that you are making the right choice for you and your baby, whatever that choice may be.

The challenge: If you are expecting or planning on starting a family make sure you get both sides of the story. Before you make any decisions book an appointment with a private (home birthing) midwife and discuss your options.

20. Set up your desk

Are you aware that the very desk that you sit at might be stressing you out? I'm not talking about your job, that annoying person you have to sit next to or even your strung-out boss. I'm talking about the actual desk!

Ideally our bodies are designed to be standing and moving around throughout the day, but your boss may not agree. One of the most prolific stresses on our bodies in our modern day lives is our posture at work. If your posture isn't right, these stressors will build up hour after hour, day after day, week after week and year after year – becoming bigger than the more obvious stressors we tend to think about. These physical stressors have also been shown to accelerate the stress response in your brain, leading you to feel emotionally stressed and even ill.

The best way to avoid this is to keep moving. Ideally you won't sit in the one place for longer than 20 minutes without moving – even if all you do is get up, do a lap around your chair and sit back down again. But for some people, even that small amount of movement is impractical. So if your job necessitates that you remain seated for lengths at a time, here are a few simple rules to help reduce your work stress. Firstly, sit up straight. This means sitting with your feet touching the floor, your knees bent to 90 degrees, hips bent to 90 degrees, and elbows at your side at 90 degrees.

The set-up of the contents of your desk is also vitally important to the stress that you put on your body. The middle of your screen should ideally be at eye-height to ensure that your head is not bent forward, and the keyboard at elbow-height to avoid strain on your shoulders. For most people this means that the chair needs to be raised or the keyboard lowered, and the screen needs to be quite a bit higher. You may also need a footrest to ensure that your feet still rest flat on the floor.

This advice can be hard to follow if you are a laptop user. If you use a laptop, get a spare keyboard for when you are in the office. Put the keyboard at the appropriate height and use the laptop as the screen. Elevate it on some phone books or a stand so that it is at the correct height.

You may not be able to do anything about the workload or the high strung boss but at least there are some work stresses that are manageable.

The challenge: Assess your work station and ensure that it is not causing postural stress to your body. Later do the same for your car and your home.

21. Focus on the long term

We have all done it. Whether it's a boozy night out or an overindulgent lunch, we have given into the temptations of now and paid for it the next day. We have a society that is based around short-term pleasure. Be it our quest for instant pain relief, crash dieting or fast food, we are constantly trying to do things easier and faster. But what are the long-term consequences?

For instance, why is it that according to one UCLA study, over two-thirds of dieters regain more weight than they lost? Or that inevitably, those people taking pain relief for their aches and pains need to keep reaching for that bottle to keep the pain away, until eventually even that doesn't give relief? And why is it that we go out for a boozy Friday night, swear in the morning that it just isn't worth it and that we will never, ever do it again, only to repeat the dose next Friday?

The reason is our short-term focus. According to life coach Anthony Robbins, we tend to make life choices around how much pleasure a certain action gives us versus how much pain that same action causes us. The problem comes when we use instant pain and pleasure as our guide. For instance, we will often make food choices based around cost, convenience and taste. These are all instant pleasures, but continually making choices based purely on these criteria will make you sick in the long term.

The solution is to make your lifestyle choices based around future pain and pleasure. When you are making a decision around anything in your life, ask yourself, 'What sort of pain will this choice potentially cause me in the future?', 'What are the long term consequences of continually doing this activity?' and 'How will this make me feel tomorrow?'.

One great way to link your food choices to long-term conse-quences is to eat your favourite junk food naked in front of the mirror. Unless you are 100 per cent happy with what you see, this can be a great reality check as to the long-term effects of what you are putting into your body! On the other hand, everyone knows that if they eat more fruits and vegetables it will mean that in the long term they will be more energetic, healthier and fitter looking.

So make your lifestyle choices based around the pleasure and pain they will cause you in the future, rather than the instant moment. You will not only be much happier and healthier but you might even start to enjoy Sunday mornings.

The challenge: For the next 21 days deliberately notice the way your lifestyle choices affect you long term and start making your health choices based on long term rather than short term effects.

22. Get more sunlight

The dangers of getting too much sun have been well documented... but did you know you can actually get *too little* sun?

It has been drummed into us for decades now that we need to avoid the sun. We have been told that over-exposure is going to cause skin cancer, leading to many of us avoiding the sun like the plague. This sun avoidance coupled with our propensity to work and play all day inside means that many people are getting precious little sunshine.

So why is getting too little sun a problem? Well as it turns out, sunlight is a vital factor in helping your body produce vitamin D, which is very important for your health. In fact vitamin D has been shown to lower the risk of many cancers, including breast and prostate cancer. It has also been associated with improvements in diabetes, depression, heart disease, arthritis, osteoporosis, infertility, fatigue, obesity and more. Pretty impressive list, huh?

So how can sunlight and vitamin D help with so many things? Well, vitamin D is not actually a vitamin – it is a precursor to steroid hormones. These fat soluble hormones are able to travel right throughout your body and affect virtually every single cell, tissue and organ.

What about sunscreen: does that make a difference? As it turns out, it does. Sunscreen can block your body's ability to produce vitamin D by up to 95 per centper cent. In fact it has been suggested that in some cases, overuse of sunscreen may be causing more cancers than it prevents.

So how much is enough and how much is too much? Of course I am not saying go out in the sun all day, nor am I encouraging sunbathing or tanning beds. But exactly how much sun you should get is hard to say because it depends on a number of factors. Like your skin tone, your latitude, the time of day, the ozone layer above you and even the levels of cloud cover and pollution.

So if you are a pale Caucasian living in Australia in the middle of summer, ten minutes in the sun may be enough. On the other hand if you are living in London in the middle of winter and have dark skin then you may be able to be exposed all day without there being any issues. When you are trying to get your vitamin D do not wear sunscreen and expose as much skin as you can. Of course if you are going to be out in the midday sun, or if your work/hobby means that you will be out in the sun all day, then the usual slip, slop, slap rules apply. Wear a hat, shirt and if you must sunscreen and protect yourself from overexposure.

It's simple as that: getting a little sun must be the most relaxing, cheapest and fun cancer prevention ever. And of course making sure you get plenty of healthy fats in your diet will help your body utilize the vitamin D fully.

The challenge: Get and extra 10 minutes of sun on your exposed skin once a week for the next 7 weeks. Attempt this challenge as many times as it takes until you are getting the appropriate amount for your specific circumstances. If you are not certain what that is ask your health care provider.

23. Remove trans fats

It turns out that when it comes to fats it is not so much how much fat you consume but what type of fat you consume that is most important. There are 'good' fats and 'bad' fats, much like 'good' cholesterol and 'bad' cholesterol. The most dangerous types of fats appear to be trans-fatty acids.

Trans fatty acids (trans-fats) are artery-clogging fats that are formed when vegetable oils are hardened into margarine or shortening. Trans-fatty acids are used instead of oil in many foods, particularly in fast food and packaged snacks such as chips, chicken nuggets and pizza, as well as bakery products including pies, doughnuts, biscuits and cakes.

Trans fats are known to increase levels of low density lipoprotein ("bad" cholesterol) in the blood, while lowering levels of high density lipoprotein ("good" cholesterol). They have also been associated with clogging of arteries, type 2 diabetes and other serious health problems including an increase the risk of heart disease.

According to the Institute of Medicine **there is no safe level of trans fats.**

While some foods like fried foods and baked goods are obvious sources of trans fats, other processed foods, such as cereals, may also contain them. One tip to determine the amount of trans-fats in a food is to read the ingredient label and look for shortening, hydrogenated or partially hydrogenated oil. The higher up on the list these ingredients appear, the more trans-fats you will be consuming.

Companies such as Nestle and Kraft have already started to make changes in the amounts of trans fats in some of their products in response to concerns about its safety and threats of litigation.

According to one study a trans fats diet reduced blood vessel function by 30 per centper cent and lowered HDL ("good")-cholesterol levels by about one fifth, compared with a saturated fats diet. Previous research has shown that trans-fats, like saturated fats, also raise LDL ("bad")-cholesterol levels. This suggests that trans-fatty acids increase the risk of heart disease much more than saturated fats.

The challenge: For the next 21 days look for trans fats in your food and remove one source from your diet. Attempt this challenge as many times as it takes until you have completely removed trans fats from your diet.

24. Say no to artificial sweeteners

When it comes to what to eat and what not to eat there is often a lot of conflicting information. One study tells you that it something is good for you whilst another tells you the exact opposite. Or all of the evidence points in one direction only to find out later that it was in fact not true.

This is almost certainly the case with diet soft drinks and artificial sweeteners in general. Have you been consuming diet soft drinks in the belief that they are a healthier option, or that they are going to help you keep your weight down?

Well, new research says that they do neither.

Aspartame and MSG are responsible for over 75per cent of all adverse reactions reported to the Food and Drug Administration (FDA) in America. They act as neurotransmitters in the brain and too much of either can cause an excessive influx of calcium into the cells, releasing free radicals that actually kill brain cells. The biggest concern with this is that three quarters of your brain cells can be killed before you notice any symptoms. Another common ingredient, Methanol Formaldehyde has also been shown to be neurotoxin whilst excessive quantities of phenylalanine has been shown to reduce the levels of the 'anti-stress' hormone serotonin in your brain. Low serotonin levels are linked to depression, strokes, cancers and diabetes.

Research also shows that low calorie products such as diet soft drinks do not help you lose weight. In fact over 10 years ago the American Cancer Society documented the fact that persons using artificial sweeteners gain more weight than those who avoid them. Artificial sweeteners have been shown to stimulate your appetite, increase your sugar cravings and stimulate storage of fat and weight gain.

The challenge: For the next 21 days remove one food containing artificial sweeteners from your diet and replace it with a healthy alternative. Attempt this challenge as many times as it takes until you have completely removed trans fats from your diet.

25. Kick pessimism

Do you believe in the mind body connection? As Deepak Chopra said to one of his colleagues, If you don't believe in the mind-body connection, how do you think that you move your finger?

There have been numerous studies that have shown a mind-body connection and one particularly has shown a link between heart disease and pessimism. A study from the Netherlands found that people that are pessimistic are more likely to die of heart disease and other causes than those who are by nature optimistic.

People with the highest level of optimism were 45 per cent less likely than those with the highest level of pessimism to die of all causes during the study. For the most optimistic, the death rate was 30.4 per cent; the most pessimistic had a death rate of 56.5 per cent. There were 397 deaths in the study, and prevention of cardiovascular mortality accounted for nearly half of the protective effects of optimism.

According to a 2002 study by Johns Hopkins researchers, angry young men are far more likely to suffer from heart attacks and cardiovascular disease before the age of 55 than their calmer counterparts. Guys who were angry in their youth were six times more likely to have a heart attack before age 55 and three times more likely to develop premature cardiovascular disease.

Up to this point there has been evidence that mental states, like depression, are linked with a significantly higher risk of cardiovascular death, but the relationship between normal personality traits like optimism and health have not been as well documented.

One of the major reasons for this link is the neurological effect of positive and negative thoughts. Every negative thought fires nerve endings in your brain that stimulate the "stress response". The stress response causes the release of adrenalin and cortisol which has a number of effects on the body and increases the risk of stroke, cancer, diabetes and heart attacks. Conversely, every positive thought has the opposite effect, helping to switch off the stress response and reduce that risk.

The challenge: Keep a diary for 2 days documenting every pessimistic thought that you have. For the following 21 days replace one of your common pessimistic thoughts with a more positive alternative. Attempt this challenge as many times as it takes until you optimistic thoughts outweigh your pessimistic ones.

26. Eat healthy meats

Human beings, as the ads say, evolved to eat red meat and in fact eating meat was an important part of our development, however we almost certainly didn't eat as much as we do in a typical western diet. Our genes have changed very little in the last 100,000 years and so our meat requirements have not changed much either. In fact there are some essential fats that we can only get in sufficient quantities by eating meat products. (EPA and DHA).

We know we are designed to eat meat, albeit less than we do now, but what is really important is the quality of the meat. There are several things that can affect its quality, such as what the cattle is fed, what hormones and drugs are used, and how the meat is cooked.

Most cattle are grain fed. I have talked before about what excessive grain consumption can do to people and it does all of the same things when fed to cattle. One of the main things that happens is that the fat ratios change. Grain-fed cattle have been shown to have more omega 6 fats that have been linked to heart disease, and less omega 3 fats which actually promote cardiac health.

Many of the cattle that are consumed also contain measurable amounts of hormones that are transferred to humans. These cows are fed a steady diet of antibiotics and hormones to help promote their growth. Amongst other things, it is believed that human consumption of oestrogen from hormone-fed beef can result in cancer, premature puberty and falling sperm counts.

If you can't find grass-fed beef, kangaroo meat is an excellent option. Kangaroo meat is lean, free range, grass-fed and organic.

But remember that overcooking, cooking on high heat and barbecuing your meat can also pose a risk. It can actually create cancer-causing substances in your food called heterocyclic amines (HCA's) and Polycyctic Aromatic Hydrocarbons (PAH's) which are potent cancer-causing agents.

So by all means enjoy your meat, but be careful of both the quality and the quantity that you consume.

The challenge: For the next 7 weeks replace one meat meal a week with lean, free range, grass fed organic meats. Attempt this challenge as many times as it takes until you only eat healthy meats.

27. Eat organic food

Is buying organic better for you?

There has been a lot of debate as to whether organic food is better for you than non-organic food. Logic tells us that we have to be better off without all of the chemicals that are associated with modern farming practices, but up until now there has been very little research to support this.

A new £12m study funded by European Union is now being prepared for publication, and the early findings are very promising for advocates of organic food. The study shows that organically produced crops and dairy milk usually contain more "beneficial compounds" such as vitamins and antioxidants than their non-organic counterparts.

The research has shown up to 40 per centper cent more beneficial compounds in vegetable crops and up to 90 per centper cent more in milk. It has also found high levels of minerals such as iron and zinc in organic produce.

Organic produce is typically about 30 per centper cent more expensive and until now people have been told that buying organic food is fine as a lifestyle choice but that there are no proven health benefits. However, this new research shows that that extra 30 per centper cent may be a very worthwhile investment.

Another study released recently and conducted by the University of California compared organic tomatoes with those grown "conventionally". It was conducted over 10 years and found double the level of flavonoids (a type of antioxidant thought to reduce the risk of heart disease) in organic food.

Don't forget though, that just because something is organic, doesn't mean that it is healthy. All of the other rules in regards to having a healthy balanced diet still apply. An organic soft drink may be healthier than a non-organic one, but it is still a soft drink.

The challenge: For the next 21 days switch a few select items of your food to organic produce. Attempt this challenge as many times as it takes until you are eating as close as possible to totally organic food.

28. Reduce your alcohol consumption

It is widely believed and talked about that drinking in moderation is good for you but there is plenty of research to indicate that this may not in fact be the case.

For instance, the *Journal of the Royal Society of Medicine* has said that "Because of the many obvious health hazards of alcohol and because the benefits of alcohol are small and ill understood the recommendation to be a light drinker is not only meaningless but also irresponsible".

Studies have shown that excessive drinking can increase your risk of getting cancer of the mouth, larynx, oesophagus, liver, colon, breast, pancreas, and lungs and according to a report from the International Agency for Research on Cancer, the more alcohol you consume, the higher your risk.

The World Health Organization has estimated that alcohol has caused over two million deaths worldwide each year and there has been shown to be a linear relationship between alcohol consumption and death over the age of 60. In other words, drink a little and be a little bit more likely to die; drink a lot and be a lot more likely.

The main benefit associated with alcohol, and especially wine, consumption is the benefit to cardiovascular health. This is largely related to the bioflavonoid and antioxidants found in the grape skins and seeds. It is not the alcohol content that is helpful.

There are better ways to get bioflavonoid and antioxidants, such as eating lots of fruits and vegetables, especially grapes.

There are also lots of other ways to improve your cardiovascular health such as eating a well balanced diet with lots of fruits, vegetables and water, eating Omega-3 fatty acids and of course exercise.

The Challenge: For one extra night a week for the next 7 weeks replace your alcoholic beverages with a healthier alternative. Attempt this as many times as it takes until you have replaced your entire alcoholic intake.

29. Start stretching

More and more Australians are suffering from spinal related health problems than ever before. In fact spinal problems affect millions of Australians and account for $4.6 billion of the nation's total health expenditure.

One of the major reasons for these problems is our sedentary lifestyles. Be it at work, at school or in the car we spend lots of time in seated postures that create stress on our spines. Stretching, flexibility and mobility exercise can be of great benefit in helping you both prevent injury and also improve performance.

A great example of this is the Straighten Up America exercise routine developed by Life University (www.straightenupamerica.org). These exercises have been designed to provide you with a simple and effective daily exercise program to improve posture and prevent spinal health problems. This simple routine helps to normalise posture, stabilise core muscle groups, enhance health and prevent spinal disability.

Straighten Up America encourages all people young and old to adopt a simple three-minute exercise program as part of their daily routine. This is the same amount of time we spend cleaning our teeth. These exercises are also great to do as a group. Be it a work or school group these exercises can be done at the start of the day, or maybe at some stage during the day to help unwind some of the stress created by our prolonged seated postures.

There are of course lots of other ways to ensure your spine is staying mobile and flexible as well. Things like yoga, Pilates and Tai Chi are fantastic ways to improve your flexibility. Doing really functional fitness is also a really good way to get your flexibility exercise at the same time as you are improving your resistance or cardiovascular fitness. A great example of this is a squat, a nice deep squat will be fantastic for improving your flexibility.

Of course if in trying these exercises you notice any restriction or pain then a visit to your local chiropractor for a check up is probably a good idea.

The challenge: One day a week for the next 7 weeks add a flexibility component to your routine. Repeat this as many times as it takes until you are doing some flexibility work each day.

30. Get a good bed and pillow

Did you know that after seven years, half of the weight of your mattress is dead skin cells? And if that isn't enough to make you want to change your mattress, there are many health concerns associated with not sleeping in the right posture, not having the right support and not getting enough sleep.

Lack of sleep has been associated with a wide range of health concerns from impaired memory and physical injuries to diabetes and cancer. It can also effect sugar and hormone balance and increase your risk of depression. A minimum amount of sleep that you should be getting is 7.5 hours – if you are getting less, it is affecting your health. Lack of sleep combined with the physical and neurological effects of having inadequate support whilst sleeping help to explain why having a good bed is really important.

To support you properly, a mattress should be as firm as is comfortable and should support you properly in all of the right areas. I always recommend people to get one a little bit firmer than they think they should in order to the best to support their spine. And remember if you have been sleeping on a softer mattress for a while it may take some time to adjust to the new firm one. Allow yourself around three weeks to adjust, and then you should be right as rain.

Choosing an appropriate pillow is also very important. I recommend getting a contoured pillow that provides support for your neck (whether you are lying on your back or on your side), and also helps to maintain the curve in your neck, which is very important for your health. You will want to make sure that the pillow is the right size as well. I always encourage my practice members to bring their pillows in to show me when they get a new one so that we can make sure that they haven't just got the right type of pillow but the right size as well.

Don't forget to look at your sleeping posture as well. The main one to avoid here is sleeping on your stomach. When you sleep on your stomach, you are effectively bending your neck to a full 90 degrees, loading it up with your body weight and then leaving it there for eight hours at a time. Over the years this adds up to be a big stress on your neck and spine.

So assess your bed, your pillow and your sleeping posture and you too can sleep your way to better health!

The challenge: Assess your bed, pillow and sleeping posture and make corrections (if necessary) to one of them. Repeat as many times as it takes until you have a healthy bed, pillow and sleeping posture.

31. Eat a healthy breakfast

People often ask me, 'If you don't drink milk or eat processed carbs and grains, then what do you eat for breakfast?'

The first thing I did was created some rules around what I wanted to get out of my breakfast.

I wanted to avoid grains, processed carbs and dairy products, which as I have outlined in other chapters, we are not designed to consume. Secondly I wanted to include lots of fruits and vegetables, especially leafy green vegetables which amongst other things help to ensure I get enough magnesium and calcium into my diet (for my bones and muscles). I also wanted to make sure that my breakfast had plenty of proteins and healthy fats, to ensure that I didn't have a big carbohydrate spike from the fruits and vegetables followed by that all-too-familiar mid-morning crash. I also realised that the healthy fats were particularly important for my brain power, enabling me to function at my best throughout the day.

So what does that leave me eating for breakfast? Well a whole range of things, things that you no doubt eat all the time. The trick is that they are not things you would usually think of as breakfast foods.

So things like cold meats (not processed meats), nuts, eggs, raw fruit and vegetables are often on my breakfast menu. The best thing about these foods is that apart from the eggs (and you can boil then before hand) there is no preparation required. They are things you can just have lying around so they are a quick easy morning snack.

I have also created my own simple breakfast that takes me around 15 minutes once a week to prepare, and then about one minute every morning to serve.

Here's what I did.

Firstly, I went out and bought (or requested for Christmas,

more precisely!) the right tools for the job: a juicer that can quickly and easily juice whole fruit, and a blender that can blend nuts fine enough so that they can be suspended in my breakfast drink. From there it is simple. Every Sunday I juice up some fresh fruit and vegetables (apples, oranges, celery, carrots or whatever you have in the cupboard at the time). Around 750 ml seems about the right amount for me. Then I add around 300 ml of water. I put this into the blender along with a large handful of nuts and two raw eggs and mix it thoroughly. Then it's done.

From there, all I need to do each morning is put the jug back on the blender for a few seconds to mix it up again, and pour it into a large glass. It's a great healthy breakfast that tastes very good (I was pleasantly surprised) and takes you very little time to make.

Of course there are plenty of other options for a healthy breakfast as well. Look for ones that are grain-free, dairy-free, made from whole foods and have a high ratio of proteins and lower carbohydrates.

The challenge: Change to a healthy grain-free, dairy-free high protein breakfast one day a week for the next 7 weeks. Repeat this challenge as many times as it takes until you are eating a healthy breakfast each and every morning.

32. Minimise antibacterial products

It seems that almost every soap and cleaner that is being brought onto the market now contains antibacterial ingredients. In fact some 72 per cent of all liquid soap sold in the United States contains them. So is this a good thing?

Are antibacterial soaps effective? Well, that depends on how you determine effective. Do they decrease the amount of bacteria on your hands or the object being cleaned? Almost certainly yes. Does this make you healthier? Almost certainly no! In fact studies have shown that people who use antibacterial soaps and cleansers get sick just as often as those who do not and in 2005 the U.S. FDA stated that there is "no added benefit" from using antimicrobial products as opposed to plain soap and water.

Not only are these soaps not helping to make you healthier, they may actually be making you sicker. Research has shown that children exposed to bacteria early in life actually have stronger immune systems whilst those who are not tend to have higher rates of both allergies and asthma. Even the American Medical Association has said that "there's no evidence that they [antibacterial soaps] do any good and there's reason to suspect that they could contribute to a problem". The other problem of course with antibacterial soaps and products is that they contribute to the formation of antibiotic-resistant bacteria, meaning that if you do get a serious infection it can be far harder to treat.

In addition, researchers have determined that about 75 per cent of a popular antimicrobial, triclocarban (TCC), resists water treatments meant to break it down and ends up in surface water. TCC is known to cause cancer and reproductive problems. Releasing these products into the environment also further adds to the development of "super-bugs".

Of course the best way to make sure that the germs in your environment aren't making you sick is to make sure that your body's resistance is as strong as possible. The only way to do this is to give your body all that it requires in terms of eating, moving and thinking.

So by all means wash your hands with soap and water, but if you want to stay healthy, avoid the antibacterial products.

The challenge: In the next 21 days replace one of your existing anti-bacterial soaps or cleaners with a non anti-bacterial one. Repeat this challenge as many times as it takes until your home is free of these products.

33. Interpret the health info

Why is it that when it comes to health there is so much conflicting information? Why is it so hard for people who are trying to take an active role in their health to get the right information?

There are two major problems with the way we are doing our health research that is leading to fundamental flaws in the answers that are being provided.

The first problem is that we are simply asking the wrong questions. One of the main reasons for this is the reductionistic way that a lot of our research is conducted. I came across a classic example of this the other day. A study had come out that had shown that things like alcohol or mobile phones did not significantly increase the chance of cancer and so should not be worried about in terms of cancer risk. What was the question that they asked? Not 'Are mobile phones good for your health?', but 'Do mobile phones by themselves cause a statistically significant increase in the cancer rates?'

The reason that this is important is that it doesn't take into account what happens if you are exposed to more than one of these stressors. It also doesn't take into account the risks of any other health conditions.

People's bodies are a complex ecosystem that has many, many variables. It simply doesn't make sense to take out all of these variables and try to study one thing in isolation; our bodies simply don't work that way.

The second fundamental problem with the way we do research is that people are not required to publish all of their research. What this means is that if I am going to fund a study into my specific drug or therapy, I can undergo as many studies as I want, tweaking the question until I get the best 'results'. I can then publish the 'best' study only, chucking the rest in the bin.

This combination of asking the wrong questions and being

selective with the answers means that virtually anything can be shown or 'proven' – not exactly a recipe for clear and concise answers that help to inform the public about what is healthy for their bodies.

Trying to keep up to date with the latest research and what it says you should do to create health is a never-ending task – especially when what we read is constantly changing and always saying different things. The best way to judge your health choices is based on what your body is designed to do – that is, to think, move and eat like our hunter-gatherer ancestors did.

The challenge: For the next 21 days ask different questions. Choose to ask 'will this make me healthier' and you will get a much better answer.

34. Consume less caffeine

Many people now realise that too much coffee is not good for you. Unfortunately, people still don't realise all of the effects. They also don't realise that many of these same effects are created by caffeinated tea and energy drinks, neither of which are in fact good for you in spite of the advertisers' claims.

Caffeine can have some positive short term benefits. It acts as a stimulant, can improve alertness and even coordination.

Unfortunately, in the long term it also has many negative side effects. The most obvious is dehydration. Caffeine acts as a diuretic, leaching valuable water that is vital for almost every cellular function in your body. Caffeine has also been shown to cause nervousness and anxiety insomnia, headaches, ulcers and reflux.

Caffeine also increases the acidity of the body. When your body is acidic it tries to neutralise it. It does this in several ways. It removes calcium from the bones (osteoporosis) and magnesium from the muscles (muscle cramps). It causes cramping of the muscles in your blood vessels leading to increased blood pressure and hence risk of heart complications and strokes.

When you body can't neutralise the acid, it stores it in your fat cells. Once the ones you have are full, your body actually creates more fat in order to safely store the acid. This increased acidity also causes increased ageing and decreased immune function.

Caffeine is particularly hazardous in pregnancy. It has been shown to increase foetal heart rate and is even linked to miscarriage.

But surely this doesn't include those "healthy" caffeinated drinks, like tea and my energy drink?

Well, these drinks may contain some healthy ingredients, like the antioxidants in tea. However you will get more than enough of these healthy ingredients by eating a diet containing lots of fruits and vegetables without all of the side effects of caffeine. Now I know that this chapter is not going to be popular with all of you caffeine addicts out there, but don't worry, I don't expect or want you to quit cold turkey. The best way to reduce your caffeine intake is to replace rather than remove.

So start to reduce your caffeine intake and you will not only start to function better you will actually find that herbal teas will open you up to a whole world of possibilities with loads of different non-caffeinated flavours to choose from.

The challenge: For the next 21 days replace one of your coffees with a tea or replace one of your teas with a low caffeine tea (green tea) or replace one of your green teas with a herbal tea. Repeat this challenge as many times as it takes until you have eliminated caffeine from your diet.

35. Become an inverse paranoid

Did you know that being optimistic can increase both your physical health and your mental functioning? For some of you this will be the bleeding obvious, and for others this will be a bit hard to swallow, and your reaction will pretty much tell you which side of the fence you sit on. Those of you who say "of course" are more than likely the optimistic ones and are already taking advantage of this fact. Those of you who say "bulldust" are more than likely the pessimistic amongst us.

Well, now it has been backed up by hard science. Research conducted by the Mayo Clinic gave 447 people a personality test in their 60s and then a health assessment in their 90s. Pessimists reported poorer physical and mental function, lower quality of life and scored lower on the eight measured scales. These results are further backed up by a previous study that showed that that optimists tend to live longer than pessimists.

How do I know if I'm a pessimist? Well one of the best ways is to simply compare yourself to those around you. Don't just pick out the ones that fit in with your preconceived ideas either. Genuinely compare yourself to everyone around you and ask yourself am I more optimistic or more pessimistic than that person. You will soon come up with your answer.

'So maybe I'm a pessimist, but that's just how I am. What can I do about it?'

Well, the first thing that you need to realise is that a pessimist isn't something you *are*, it is something you *do*. It may have become such an ingrained habit that you now do it unconsciously but it is still something you can change. One of the best examples of how to do this is the author W Clement Stone. He *chose* to believe that the whole world was conspiring to help him. This is what he called being an 'inverse paranoid'. This means that whenever something he perceived as good happened to him, he said thanks. Whenever something that other people perceived as bad happened he said thanks, with the understanding that it had happened to teach him a lesson or provide an opportunity that would make his life better in the long run.

The challenge: For the next 21 days look for the opportunity in every challenge and start choosing to believe that the universe is conspiring to help you.

36. Eat less salt

Most people by now have a fair idea that too much salt is bad for you. What they often do not realise though is what contains salt and how bad it is.

The average diet contains around 10 grams of salt per day. That is 4 grams of sodium and 6 grams of chlorine.

Eating too much sodium has long been linked to high blood pressure and heart disease but there are many other adverse effects that are often not considered. However one of the biggest factors is not the sodium, but the chloride. Chloride, as with many other elements of our western diets raises the body's acidity. Acidity causes many adverse effects in your body including osteoporosis, muscle spasms, increased blood pressure, heart disease, stroke, kidney stones, asthma, stomach cancer and insomnia. In fact too much acidity in your diet affects virtually every aspect of your health and vitality.

Most people also don't realise that most of the salt you eat comes not from the shaker on the table but from the processed foods that you are eating. Foods like canned soups, cheeses, bacon, hot dogs and processed meats, sauce and gravy mixes, stuffing, soy sauce, bread and many other processed foods contain much more salt than we are designed to eat.

So when it comes to lowering your salt intake it really pays to keep it simple. Simple unprocessed foods are the key, fruits and vegetables, water, healthy unsalted nuts and healthy unsalted meats. Remember that is takes 21 days to break a habit and it may take that long to get used to the real taste of your food without the salt, so be sure to give it a little time, you will be glad you did.

The challenge: Start reading your food labels and being aware of how much salt you are adding to home cooked meals. For the next 21 days remove one source of excess salt from your diet. Repeat as many times as it takes until you have are having no more than a pinch of sea salt a say.

37. Allocate some 'me time'

Are you stressing your way to cancer? A new report illustrates how the stress hormone norepinephrine accelerates the formation of tumours and facilitates the growth of existing tumours. As evidence mounts showing the chronic health effects of stress from cancers to strokes, and heart disease to diabetes, it has become more and more obvious that stress minimisation is vital for health and wellbeing.

Now usually when I talk to one of my friends about stress minimisation they roll their eyes look at me like the latent hippie that I am but it need not be so weird. Meditation, yoga and reiki may not be for everyone, but the good news is that they don't need to be. In order to de-stress your life, all you need to do is find a healthy activity that you enjoy doing – and that makes you feel relaxed.

For me, this might mean going for a walk, playing cricket, reading a book or going fishing, but for you it might mean something totally different.

Remember though, there are many things that stimulate the stress response in your body, including poor food choices, poor postures, stressful physical activities and thought patterns. So make sure that whatever you are doing to try and reduce stress isn't actually inadvertently creating more of it! This means that gorging on a chocolate cake because it makes you feel good is out, as is sitting in front of the TV for an entire day.

The most important part of this process is to make sure that you schedule some time to de-stress. It can't be something that you try to do if you 'get time', because for most people that time will never come. You need to set a special time aside, without interruptions, where you can totally and fully relax.

So turn off the mobile, leave the laptop at home and just relax. You will not only feel better, but you will be healthier too.

The challenge: For the next 7 weeks create a regular time in your week when you do something healthy for you that allows you to relax.

38. Eat local

Locavore; one who eats locally

If you haven't been to your local farmers market (they are springing up everywhere) here are a few reasons that you should.

1. **The economy.** Who doesn't want to support our local farmers? We all have an affinity with the man on the land. The money we spend on their produce all goes back to the local community. These farmers shop at our shops, eat at our restaurants and use our local services.
2. **Fresh is best.** We all know that fresh food is better for us, not to mention tastier. Food at your local farmers market may be only days or even hours old, whereas fruit in your local supermarket may have been in cold store for much longer, losing nutrients and vitality along the way.
3. **In season.** Ayurvedic and Chinese doctors have been advocating eating what is in season for thousands of years and of course our hunter gatherer ancestors had no choice. So it makes sense that we have evolved to require whatever is in season at that point in time and by doing so we ensure that we get a good range of healthy fresh food.
4. **Less processed.** One of the biggest issues we face at the moment is the fact that we don't eat enough real food. Too much of our food has additives, sweeteners, preservatives and chemicals and each of these has its own adverse health effects.
5. **Better for the environment.** We all want to reduce our environmental footprint and what easier way to do that than to eat local. This means that the food transportation is down and therefore it is less polluting for the environment.
6. **More informed.** One of the keys to living a healthy life is to be well informed. One of the best things about a farmers

market is that you can go there and either talk to the farmer or someone closely involved in the farm and find out everything you want to know. Is it genetically modified, is it sprayed, it is organic and do they use sustainable farming practices?

The challenge: In the next 21 days check out your local farmers market and purchase some fresh, in-season, unprocessed, healthy, organic produce.

39. Eat more fibre

Research from the International Journal of Cancersuggests that men can lower their risk of prostate cancer by eating vegetables. More than 1,700 men were studied (with and without prostate cancer) who consumed fibre mainly from vegetable sources, and showed a decrease in their prostate cancer risk. In fact men who consumed most of their fibre from vegetables were 18 per cent less likely to develop prostate cancer, whereas those who received their fibre from fruits or grains didn't show a decrease in prostate cancer risks. Obviously vegetables have many other benefits as well, including preventing heart disease, other cancers, diabetes etc.

When I tell people that I don't eat breads, processed carbs or grains, they often ask me, 'What about fibre?' The truth of the matter is that you can get all of the fibre you need by eating enough fruits and vegetables. In fact the fibre that you get from eating loads of good quality fruits and vegetables is actually much better for you, as the above study has shown.

Combine that with the fact that you don't get the negative health effects of the processed carbs and the fact that those fruits and veggies provide loads of other health benefits, and it is really a no brainer.

So eat lots of fruits and vegetables as part of your balanced diet and you will be well on your way to reducing your prostate cancer risk. And remember, the reason to eat your veggies is not to reduce your prostate cancer risk – it is to make your body healthy. Having an appropriate weight, better performance, better moods and reduced risk of disease are all simply side effects of having a healthy body.

The Challenge: Eat one extra serve of vegetables each day for the next 21 days. Repeat as many times as it takes until you are eating 8-9 serves of vegetables a day

40. Incorporate some balance exercise

Many people's exercise routines are missing one key ingredient: balance. And I don't just mean that they are not doing a diverse enough routine – I mean that they don't include activities that test their ability to keep their balance.

So why is keeping your balance so important? Well for a start, falls are the leading cause of death for those over the age of 60 years. So as you get older, keeping your balance becomes very important. But balance isn't just important for preventing falls. The key ingredient for keeping your balance is the feedback you get from your body. It's called proprioception, and is essentially your body's awareness of where it is in space. The better quality your proprioceptive feedback, the easier it is to stay on your own two feet.

It turns out that proprioception is important for much more than just keeping your balance. Proprioceptive feedback to your brain has been shown to stimulate the release of dopamine and serotonin – our body's "feel good" chemicals. Their release helps to switch off your body's stress response, which has been linked to chronic diseases like strokes, cancers, heart disease and diabetes. Switching off your stress response has also been shown to increase the function of your immune system, improve your concentration, help normalise your cholesterol profile and much more.

How do you incorporate balance into your exercise routine? Well obviously utilising a class like yoga or body balance would be a great way to start. Or at home, an exercise routine like the 'Straighten Up Australia' program designed by the Chiropractors Association of Australia can be a very simple way to introduce some basic balance work into your day. If these seem a little mundane for you there are some more physical options too. Activities like squats, Olympic lifts and gymnastic exercises such as headstands can all help to improve your balance and stimulate your proprioception. Of course remember that when it comes to proprioception, it is the quality of movement that is key, so if you have restricted movement, particularly in your spine, getting a check up with a chiropractor can be of added benefit.

Is your lack of balance putting your health off balance?

The challenge: At least once a week for the next 7 weeks incorporate some activity that requires balance into your exercise routine. Repeat this challenge as many times as it takes until you are doing this regularly once a day.

41. Be informed on vaccination

I have no doubt that this will be the most popular (and the most inflammatory) chapter in this book. Any time I speak out about vaccination it seems to stir up a real hornet's nest. The reason is that vaccination is a very personal issue, and one that is prone to very severe biases (from both sides of the agenda). Because of these biases, it can be very hard to figure out the truth. If you listen to the pro-vaccination lobby, you would swear that it is the best thing since sliced bread and that not vaccinating should be illegal! If you listen to the anti-vaccination groups, they will tell you that vaccines and vaccine manufacturers are pure evil and that they are killing and maiming our children in order to make a profit. The truth is most likely somewhere in between.

Firstly let me say that the principle behind vaccination is very sound. The best defence you have against almost any disease is your own body and your own immune system. Of course vaccines have side-effects as well – even the most ardent vaccine supporter will not argue with that – so the question then becomes, do the positives outweigh the negatives? Are we sure? And are there safer, cheaper and more effective ways to boost our immune system? If it can be shown that the benefits of vaccines outweigh the negatives, then yes, getting shots would be a good idea.

What we don't have is long-term, double-blind, randomised control studies comparing vaccinated and non-vaccinated groups – and we probably never will. Despite this being the gold standard in medical research, we have never had this type of research done, because vaccine supporters claim that it would be 'unethical' to not vaccinate a group of people, in spite of the fact that many people (including a significant portion of doctors) choose not to vaccinate.

So we are left looking at population studies. People will often look at population studies showing a reduction in rates of communicable diseases and suggest that the reduction since the advent of the vaccine is proof of efficacy. However when you look at stats going back further, you realise that many of these communicable diseases had been on decline well before the introduction of the vaccine. The reductions were in fact more closely associated with cleaner water, better living conditions, improved sanitation and improved nutrition than they were to vaccination.

So the benefits may not be as significant as we have been led to believe. But what about the risks? One thing you need to remember when analysing the risk / benefit of vaccination is the fact that adverse vaccine reactions are severely under-reported – so much so that studies have reported that only 1-10 per centper cent of vaccine reactions are ever actually reported. Think about it: that means that whenever you read about vaccine side-effects, you need to multiply the numbers by 10 to 100 times to get a true indication. This all starts to alter the cost / benefit equation a bit, doesn't it?

'If I don't get the vaccine, won't I be putting my friends and family at risk?'

Well, not if the vaccine works. If the vaccine is as effective as people claim, then surely a vaccinated person would have no need to fear you at all...? Remember also that just because someone is vaccinated does not mean that they are not able to carry and spread the disease. A vaccine helps your body to fight off the disease – it DOES NOT prevent you from getting it or carrying it. In fact a recent study that asked whether vaccinating healthcare workers helped to protect the elderly they were looking after showed that it made no difference to the patients' health outcomes.

So remember, we each have the right to accept or decline vaccinations based on our own informed decisions. I encourage you to do some research, investigate BOTH the pros and the cons and make a decision that sits comfortably with you and your family. If you do this, you will have made the right decision for you.

The challenge: Investigate before you vaccinate. Seek out both sides of the vaccine story and be sure that the decision you are making is the best one for YOU and YOUR FAMILY.

42. Keep your healthy probiotics

If you haven't heard about Probiotics by now you must have been living under a rock. It seems every day we are bombarded with new info and new ads promoting the latest beneficial bacteria. What always amuses me is that it is usually right after the latest anti-bacterial soap ad claiming to kill even more of those "little nasties". So what is the story – are bacteria good or bad? Do we want to kill them or swallow them?

The truth is that a healthy body has a good balance of different bacteria. Your gut contains over a kilogram of bacteria (that's over 100 trillion cells). These bacteria naturally keep each other in check and work with your body's immune system to make it harder for "bad" bacteria to invade. They also help to digest food and even produce some nutrients that our bodies cannot make themselves.

So why have Probiotics become so important all of a sudden? I mean, what did people do before they could buy their bacteria in yoghurt or tablet form? Well, they got their bacteria from their environment and even more importantly, once their gut had been colonised by a good balance of healthy bacteria, they didn't kill them off!

Not killing your bacteria off is the key. Many of our modern lifestyle choices are either killing off or unbalancing our natural bacterial flora. Our high sugar, high processed carbohydrate diets overfeed the bacteria living inside us, leading to a disruption of the natural healthy balance. Other lifestyle choices such as alcohol consumption, antibiotics, the contraceptive pill and other medications will actually kill off your natural healthy bacterial colonies.

If you have a healthy diet and lifestyle and don't drink or take antibiotics, your stomach will find its own healthy balance. If it doesn't – and/or if you are experiencing bloating, gas, or discomfort – then it might be worthwhile giving some of those commercially available Probiotics a go for up to 30 days. If it still doesn't resolve consult your health care provider.

The challenge: Only take antibiotics when they are absolutely necessary. If necessary try a Probiotics supplement for up to 30 days and consult your health care provider.

43. Check your nervous system

More and more people are really starting to jump onto the wellness revolution. Everywhere I look now there are people talking and reading about diet, exercise and positive thinking, and it is fantastic. However, there is one key link that many people are missing – which links all of these things together and controls every cell, tissue and organ in your body.

'My brain?' you say. Well, you're close. But I want you to think of your brain like a computer. Now if you don't touch your computer, what will it do? That's right, nothing. It has all of the information there, but until it receives some input, you won't get any output. Your brain is just the same. It needs input from your internal and external environment before it can give any output. This input comes via your nervous system.

The thing that many people are missing is that if you are eating, thinking and moving in a very healthy way, but your nervous system is not processing it healthily, then you are not going to receive their full benefits.

Think of it this way. If you're getting lots and lots of fantastic vitamins in your healthy diet, but your nervous system supplying your gut isn't functioning properly, are you going to get the full benefit of those vitamins? Well, probably not, because if your gut isn't getting the right messages, it may not produce the right chemicals to help you digest and absorb those nutrients.

Why would there be interference to your nervous system? Well, stress basically: physical, chemical and emotional stressors such as poor posture or constant tension can cause a misalignment or restriction to one of the vertebrae in your spine (a subluxation). Left untreated, this will cause interference to your nervous system and hinder all of those well-intended lifestyle efforts you are making.

So what is the answer? If you feel like you've been making the necessary lifestyle changes but haven't been getting the results you want to see (or even if you have), perhaps it's time to get your nervous system checked by a chiropractor.

The challenge: If you haven't done so already in the next 21 days get a check up from a Chiropractor.

44. Don't fall for marketing spin

Healthy is the new buzz word: everyone wants their products to be associated with health benefits. The simple way to 'spin' this is to find one ingredient in your product (if you can't find one, add one) that can be clinically shown to be healthy, then promote it like crazy: coffee 'with anti-oxidants', sugary cereals 'with vitamin B', dairy products 'with calcium', soft drinks 'with real lemon'. Then there are the low-fat products that fail to mention that they contain loads of fattening sugar.

These clever marketers take advantage of our reductionist scientific method. We take one small part of the product (calcium) and we do a study to see how it affects one small part of our body (our bones). We then take the health benefits we see and extrapolate them to say that that means the whole product is healthy for the whole body. To show how ridiculous this is, let's use an extreme example: if I add antioxidants to arsenic, will it make it healthy?

There are loads of unhealthy products, from coffee to chocolate to alcohol to sugary drinks, which claim to be healthy because they contain high levels of anti-oxidants. The thing is, there is no health advantage to eating more anti-oxidants than your body needs. And if you eat sufficient fruits and vegetables, you will not only get as many anti-oxidants as you need, you will also get many, many more nutrients that your body vitally needs. Fruits and vegetables also won't create side-effects in your body that reduce your capacity to utilise the vitamins you are taking in.

What this means is that if you are eating your fruits and vegetables, the anti-oxidants in these unhealthy products are providing no real benefit – so only the negative effects remain.

Similarly there are plenty of products on the shelf with titles like 'high energy' and 'low fat' that try to insinuate that they are great for you. If you unravel the spin however, what they are really saying is that they are really high in sugar. We all know that sugary foods are bad for us and that in the long run they will give us less energy not more.

So don't fall for the marketing spin! Eat a balanced, healthy diet and you'll get all the nutrients (and anti-oxidants) you need.

The challenge: For the next 21 days examine the marketing spin all around you more carefully. Ask yourself the question, 'will this make my whole body healthier?'.

45. Allow time for unwinding

Have you ever started a new health regime and noticed that you felt worse before you felt better? This is a process that I like to call unwinding.

A perfect example is when you start a new intensive exercise regime. It often feels really hard while you are doing it and you may feel sore for days or even weeks after that first session. Does that mean that the exercise is bad for you? Probably not. It just means that you have used your body in a way that it hasn't experienced in a while, and it isn't used to it.

What actually happens is that in order to make new muscle cells, the old cells are damaged and destroyed. Sounds bad, doesn't it? But actually, it's good because these are then replaced by new stronger muscle cells that are better able to meet the new demands you are putting on your body.

Similarly when you start a new diet, a new therapy (such as chiropractic) or even start changing your thought patterns, it may initially be hard. During this part of unwinding you may feel sore, anxious and depressed because the increased pressure leads you to think you're getting worse – but you may not be!

Of course you should consult with your health care professional to make sure that you aren't doing the wrong thing. But you should not automatically assume that it is therefore bad for you. In fact those very same symptoms may be a sign that you are on the right track. As your body unwinds, these symptoms tell you that things are changing – and isn't that why you started your new regime in the first place?

We are conditioned in our modern society that all symptoms are bad and that we should do whatever it takes to avoid them, but sometimes some short-term aches and pains can reap a massive long-term gain in terms of your health.

So remember, when the going gets tough, the tough get

healthy!

The challenge: Don't give up when the going gets tough. Give your body a chance to unwind when you start a new health challenge.

46. Be aware of your perception

A study of over 6,000 British civil servants has determined that people who perceive they have been treated unfairly are more likely to suffer a heart attack or chest pain. In fact those who believed they had experienced the worst injustice were 55 per cent more likely to experience a coronary event than people who thought life was fair.

Participants were asked how strongly they agreed with the statement, "I often have the feeling that I am being treated unfairly," after which they were tracked for almost 11 years, on average.

Are there things in your life that you perceive as injustices? Thoughts that you have been hanging on to for a while? Well they could be making you sick.

What's more these events you have been hanging onto may not even have been totally negative things. In fact often the things we perceive as being negative are really just that, a perception. Now I know what you are saying, but my stuff was definitely negative! Well have you really analysed it to be sure that is true or are you just judging it based on your perceptions and emotional responses. I mean if Nelson Mandela can find positives in being jailed for all those years, then maybe you can at least feel less negative about your situation.

Well here is a tool to help you find out. It is really simple, make four columns. In the first column write the negative aspects of your particular situation. Take your time, make it as long as possible. Now in the second column write the positive things about the same situation. This might be harder but take your time, you will be surprised how many there are, in fact you need to make this column as long as the first (this bit isn't easy but bear with it). Now in the third column write all the positives of that situation never having happened at all. Now in the final column, write all the negatives of the situation never happening.

What you will find is that once you have written out these four lists your level of injustice will feel lower. The cool thing about this is that it also means your level of health will be higher.

The Challenge: Pick the one thing that you are most pessimistic about and use this perception tool to help break it down.

47. Focus on getting healthy

So often I have people asking me 'What is the best way to lose weight? What is the best way to get more energy? What is the best way to optimise my sports performance? What is the best way to sleep better or to de-stress?'

The funny thing is, the answer to all of these things is exactly the same. You should not focus on trying to change any of these things, you should focus on getting healthy and everything else will follow.

After all, there are plenty of unhealthy ways to lose weight; there are plenty of unhealthy ways to sleep better or to improve your sports performance. The problem with all of these, though, is that whilst you may solve one problem, you will often create many others.

No matter what is going on in your body you will benefit from eating a healthy diet, getting some regular well-rounded exercise, thinking some healthy positive thoughts and ensuring there is no interference to your nervous system. If you do all of these things well, then everything else will take care of itself. You will sleep better, have fewer injuries, find a healthy weight and much, much more.

So start changing your goals: rather than focusing on what you want to get rid of focus on what you can do, and start making real, long-lasting changes to your health and your quality of life.

The challenge: For the next 21 days focus on what will make you healthier not what will make you skinnier, musclier, fitter, more energetic etc. etc. Repeat this challenge as many times as it takes until this way of thinking is the norm.

48. Exercise intensity

Have you ever been to a gym and watched all those people strolling along on a treadmill, reading a magazine and chatting away without missing a beat, and wondered 'Is that all it takes to get fit?'

Well it turns out that if you want to be really fit and healthy, a little more effort and intensity is required. Research shows that the intensity of the exercise you do is just as important as the type of exercise or the technique. Often public awareness programs focus on making sure people get regular low intensity exercise, primarily because it helps with weight loss, the latest hot topic. However this fat burning exercise is only one part of the whole picture.

Well-rounded exercise really is the key if you want to be truly fit – and more importantly, healthy. Combining your low intensity (endurance) exercise with some higher intensity (interval) training will help you get much better results. In fact one study from the *Journal of Applied Physiology* showed that people could actually increase their endurance by utilising higher intensity workouts. Another study published in the same journal showed that interval training leads to 36per cent better fat burning and 13per cent better cardiovascular (heart) fitness. In fact, adding some higher intensity interval training to your workout helps you to burn more fat, even when you return to lower intensity exercise.

So what is interval training?

Put simply, it means short bursts of high intensity exercise, from 30 seconds to a few minutes. It needs to be high enough intensity to get you out of breath. This is then followed by a short rest period or what is called partial recovery. In other words, it should not be long enough for you to fully return to resting heart rate. A good guide is about half of the length of time you are exercising for, then repeat several times.

One great example of high intensity exercise is the Tabata Protocol. Named after a Japanese researcher and was developed by the head coach of the Japanese speed skating team. It involves doing 20 seconds of intense activity followed by 10 seconds of rest. To start with you may only be able to do four rounds of this if you are working hard enough, however as you go along you should be able to work up to seven rounds. Even allowing for a warm-up and a warm-down, this means it will only take 15 minutes for your workout. The type of activity doesn't really matter so you can do this with sprints, cycling, rowing or even squats.

The key difference between Tabata and regular interval training is the shorter recovery time. This 'partial' recovery means that the heart and lungs are working harder. Working your heart and lungs hard is a really important part of your exercise routine and also your overall health. Think of your heart and lungs like any other muscle in your body: the harder you work them, the stronger they get – and the stronger they get, the more able they are to deal with the stresses of everyday life.

Working out using a combination of low intensity, longer workouts and higher intensity, shorter workouts will ensure that your body is more adaptable and therefore healthier, not to mention fitter and more toned.

The challenge: Incorporate some high intensity interval training into your exercise routine one day a week for the next 7 weeks. Repeat this challenge as many times as it takes until you are doing interval training several times a week.

49. Get some resistance exercise

When it comes to health and wellness, resistance exercise is a funny one. Many people think that you only need to do resistance exercise if you want to have abs to show off to the world, or you want to be an elite sportsperson. In fact even the recommendations from doctors and government agencies will suggest that a half hour walk or run a day is all you need to stay fit and healthy. But the reality is that we all need to be doing well-rounded exercise, including some resistance, if we want to be healthy and well.

Resistance exercise helps to:

- Increase muscle strength, power, endurance and size
- Increase bone density and strength
- Reduce body fat
- Increase muscle-to-fat ratio
- Boost metabolism (burning more kilojoules when at rest)
- Lower heart rate and blood pressure after exercise (thought to reduce the risk of heart disease)
- Improve balance and stability
- Enhance performance of everyday tasks
- Reduce risk of, and lead to improvement of, medical conditions – for example, diabetes (NIDDM) and arthritis

In fact many people don't realise that resistance exercise will have a bigger impact on your bone density than dietary changes will. So don't fall into the trap of thinking that cardiovascular exercise alone will make you fit and healthy. We often hold up endurance athletes like marathon runners as 'the fittest people in the world', but in reality they would be unable to complete some of the simplest resistance exercise routines. You will also find that resistance exercise will have immediate benefits in terms of your daily activities. You will find that your daily tasks become easier, you will have more energy, better posture and you will feel and look great.

Of course when you are doing resistance exercise it is important to do it right. Technique is vital when it comes to resistance training, so you may want to get a personal trainer to help make sure you are not doing yourself more harm than good. And if you are going to be putting this sort of strain on your body then you will want to be sure it is well aligned and functioning properly too, so a check-up with your local chiropractor might be in. People often forget that you are doing resistance exercise every day, like when you pick up those heavy bags of shopping. Learning how to do it right can save you many problems later on.

And remember: you don't need to be doing Olympic lifting to get some resistance exercise. The key is to start small and gradually work your way up. You can get resistance exercise by swimming in a pool, doing aquarobics, taking a class at your gym or even doing simple exercises at home. Whatever you do, start including some resistance exercise into your routine and you will quickly realise what you have been missing out on.

The challenge: Once a week for the next 7 weeks add a half hour routine of resistance exercise to your routine. Repeat this challenge as many times as it takes until you are doing resistance exercise 2-3 times a week.

50. Do some cardio exercise

There is a lot of confusion nowadays about cardiovascular (endurance) exercise. Some people will say that it is the be-all and end-all, whilst others say that we don't even need to do it at all. And as is often the case, the truth is somewhere in the middle.

There is no doubt that our bodies are made to move. We are not designed to be anywhere near as stationary as we are in our modern lives, and as a result we now have to actually work hard to achieve cardiovascular fitness (which would have been part of daily life for our ancestors). In fact I read one study recently that said that even our country cousins on the farm are now not getting enough daily exercise since the advent of modern machinery.

So what are the benefits of 'cardio' exercise? Well, it helps to maintain your weight, strengthen your heart and lungs, reduce stress, reduce disease risk, improve your moods, sleep better and have more energy. Sounds like fun, huh?

So how often should you be doing some cardiovascular exercise? Every day! You should be incorporating cardio into both your daily exercise routine and also your daily life. This doesn't mean you can only do long runs or walks, either. You can actually improve your cardiovascular fitness by doing a high intensity weights session, or by doing interval training. You can also improve your cardiovascular fitness by walking to work or taking the stairs, so have some fun with it and keep varying your routine. It will help you avoid boredom, it will keep you motivated and it will give you a more well-rounded fitness base.

Start taking every opportunity to improve your cardiovascular fitness, and remember it is not the be-all and end-all – in fact it is only one of nine components of a healthy exercise routine.

The Challenge: Once a week for the next 7 weeks add half an hour extra cardiovascular exercise to your routine. Repeat this challenge as many times as it takes until you are doing at least half an hour of 'cardio' a day.

51. Minimise medications

People who regularly read my columns or website will know that I often talk about the side effects of different treatments. I also spend a lot of time talking about prevention and lifestyle as a way of avoiding medical care. Many people infer from this that I am against all forms of modern medicine and so when I took last week off to go under a general anaesthetic and have my wisdom teeth out I got a few strange looks from my regular clients.

What people need to understand is that I am not against medical care, I am against unnecessary medical care. In our modern society much of the care people are receiving is either for entirely preventable diseases or is merely masking a much bigger problem.

I like to refer to our current medical model as a crisis care model, because drugs and surgery can be of amazing benefit when you get to the crisis stage. If you have let your lifestyle go to the point that you now have a life-threatening disease, or perhaps you have had a one-off traumatic event that is no fault of your own, then doctors can do amazing things. If I was ever to be having a heart attack I know where I would head (and it wouldn't be to my local chiropractor). So when my teeth had gotten to the point that they were causing issues and one had even cracked, I knew it was time to get something done.

Having said that, I still felt it was my responsibility to minimise the effects of the medications on my body as much as possible. In hospital I let the doctors do their work and took what they requested I take (they assured me it wasn't possible without drugs). I was then given some pain killers and instructions on when to take them and headed off home. My decision was to minimise my medications as much as possible (the drugs I was given in hospital were in fact the first medications I had taken in over 12 years). I knew that the drugs were serving no purpose other than pain control, so I knew it was perfectly safe to not follow orders in this case. So instead of popping the first pill before the general wore off as requested, I decided to wait and see how bad it was, to see whether I really needed that drug (and its side effects).

What I found to my surprise was that the pain wasn't that bad and that with some rest and a little ice to reduce the swelling, it was more than manageable. I also ensured that I drunk as much water as possible, tried to eat as healthily as I could (though there are limited options when you can't chew and can barely swallow!), got plenty of rest and returned to exercise as soon as I could. All of these things helped ensure that my body would process the toxins I had been given as quickly as possible.

So there are times when drugs and surgery can be very useful. But always remember that wellness is an active, life-long process. By eating, thinking and moving in a healthy way you can greatly reduce the need for drugs and surgery in your life. And even when you do go down that path, it is still your responsibility to minimise the traumatic effects as much as you possibly can (consulting with your doctor of course). So look after your body – it is the only one you have – and do everything you can to reduce the need for drugs and surgery.

The challenge: Be active when it comes to your intake of medication. Ask lots of questions and in the next 21 days find out which drugs are absolutely necessary and what you can do to reduce the need for them in the short and long term.

52. Use healthy cooking oils

Given all of the research that is coming out about the dangers of trans fats (hydrogenated oils) and their link to chronic disease many people are reconsidering which oils they use in their cooking. Olive oil is one healthy option that many people are turning to. However what many people don't realise is that whilst olive oil is very healthy when you are not heating the food it can be damaged by heat. In fact, when heated olive oil produces chemicals that have been linked to breast cancer and heart disease.

So what is left?

Well as it turns out one of the healthiest oils to cook with in coconut oil. Coconut oil was previously assumed to be unhealthy due to the high levels of saturated fats however we now realise that saturated fat is not the evil it was made out to be and is certainly healthier than trans-fats. These saturated fats make coconut oil much less susceptible to damage when it is heated.

So anytime you need an oil to cook with, coconut oil can replace butter, margarine, olive oil or any other type of oil in your recipes. Of course organic coconut oils are the best as they have not been refined, bleached or deodorised.

The Challenge: In the next 21 days source and buy a jar of coconut oil.

53. Stop smoking

Did you know that a review of hundreds of studies into smoking cessation by a Sydney University team has revealed that up to three quarters of ex-smokers gave up without resorting to nicotine replacement therapies?

Yeah that's right, old-fashioned willpower alone was enough to make them quit their habit. Not only that, but the studies that do show the benefit of patches, gums and pills are more than twice as likely to have been funded by drug companies. In fact in the independent studies only 22per cent found patches and gums to be of significant benefit. Makes you think, doesn't it?

So just like pretty much every other healthy change you want to make, when it comes to quitting, the will to do it and the discipline to follow through are the two most important tools you have. Remember the rules of goal setting as well: you will probably not be successful if you 'try and quit' or 'give it a go' – you are much more likely to succeed if you 'decide to become a non-smoker'. Semantics I know, but trust me, it makes a difference.

Don't get me wrong. I am not saying that quitting smoking will be easy. It won't. But it will be rewarding. In fact, probably more rewarding than any other health change you make. Why is that? Well, when you give up smoking you don't just look and feel healthier (eventually), you also save lots and lots of money.

It is really important when you quit to keep reminding yourself of the hazards of smoking and the benefits of quitting. One of the best ways to keep reminding yourself of the benefits of quitting is to place all the money that you would have spent on cigarettes into a separate bank account. Label it 'Holidays' (or 'New car' or whatever it is that you really want) and watch the money grow. Also, create a hard and fast rule for yourself: you are only allowed to buy that dream holiday if you stay off the smokes. Check your bank account regularly and each time you do, remind yourself of the benefit you are getting.

Give up smoking today. That's right: not tomorrow, or next week, or after you finish this pack. There has never been a better time than right now and you have all the tools to do it right there in your brain. Your body and your bank balance will thank you for it!

The Challenge: for the next 21 days decide to BE a non smoker.

54. Exercise accurately

One skill that is often overlooked in your average exercise routine is accuracy. Now accuracy sounds like something you would only need out on a sporting field – do you really need it in your fitness regime? I mean, if you're not an Olympic basketballer or an AFL footballer, does it really matter how accurate you are? Well as it turns out, it does, and here's why.

When you are attempting to move accurately you rely on a few things. Firstly, feedback from your body about where it is in space, then accurate transmission of those messages from your body to your brain, and finally an appropriate reaction from your body.

As it turns out, that feedback from your body about where it is in space is very important for your brain and for your health. It is called 'proprioception' and these messages have been likened to the wind that drives the windmill when it comes to brain function. The more you can exercise this feedback, be it from balance or from accuracy training, the better your brain will function, the healthier and less stressed you will be.

The accurate transmission is also very important. Whilst not necessarily something that can be improved via exercise, if there is interference to the nervous system it may mean that you are not getting the full benefit from your exercise. If you think you may have some interference in this area, or would like to find out if you do, it might be time for a check up with a chiropractor.

Finally, the appropriate bodily response: in order for your body to do something accurately you need to utilise your fine muscle control and your intrinsic muscles. This means that you need to not only learn how to move something with force, but also with control. Having this fine control of your muscle fibres becomes really important when it comes to injure prevention as well as movement efficiency.

So what sorts of things can you do to add accuracy to your exercise routine? Well the good news is that things that involve accuracy are usually pretty fun – be it sports, throwing and catching a ball (against a wall if necessary) or dribbling a soccer ball between cones. In fact there are limitless ways that you can add some accuracy to your exercise routine, so have a play with it and see what you can come up with.

Have fun!

The Challenge: For the next 7 weeks ensure your exercise routine contains something that challenges your accuracy at least once a week.

55. Don't feel guilty

I have never been a massive Rugby fan but former Wallabies captain John Eales has my favourite ever sporting nickname. They used to call him Nobody, because he was always so perfect (i.e. nobody's perfect). It is true in all things in life, including our lifestyles. Nobody is going to eat exactly the right things all the time, nobody is going to exercise perfectly, and nobody is free of negative thoughts. And it is how you think about and deal with these occasional imperfections that will decide how healthy you become. Do you treat these moments as an earned reward or a moment of learning?

Some people will see a break from their healthy routine as a reward to be savoured; as a special celebration. The problem with this is that is sets up a connection in your brain. You learn to associate unhealthy behaviours with the best times in your life. This is why some people resort to over-eating or drinking in times of stress. They associate these behaviours with having fun, an escape and a celebration, and they mistakenly believe that it will make them feel better. And in the short term, it often does. If repeated in the longer term though, it will lead to poor health, increased stress, unhappy moods and, often, guilt.

Now as I have already stated, nobody is perfect, so there is absolutely no reason to feel guilty about slipping up – everyone does it. The key is to use it as a tool to help you do better next time. Instead of focusing on how you feel at the time, start to focus on how you feel afterwards. Start to focus on how those actions make you look, feel and act. What you will begin to realise is that whilst unhealthy behaviours may have a short term positive impact on you, they will definitely have a very real, longer term negative impact. And the more you pay attention to it and notice it, the more it will start to impact your future decision making.

You will find that next time you reach for that cream bun you will remember how tired you felt last time you ate too much junk food and how good you were feeling when you started to eat a little healthier. And you will make a healthier choice – not out of guilt or fear, but as a positive choice based around creating a happier healthier life. Best of all, you will feel great for it.

The Challenge: For the next 21 days choose to perceive your 'set backs' as learning opportunities and make the most of the lessons learnt. Don't feel guilty.

56. Reduce repetitive micro-trauma

People often come in to see me in my practice and are astounded at how poorly their body is functioning. Often they want to link their current problems to some recent traumatic event that may have caused it – and just as often, that event doesn't exist.

People frequently tell me "I just woke up like this", "it came on out of nowhere" or "I just bent down to pick up a pen". Now obviously these incidents have not caused their significant dysfunction. So what is the cause? Well, often it comes down to what I call repetitive micro-trauma. In other words rather than being one big event, it may be lots of little stressors building up over a lifetime.

So what are these repetitive stresses? Well they can be virtually anything that you do repeatedly over a period of time. For some people it is their posture sitting at their computer, for others it might be shovelling sand, or kids studying at a desk. For me it might be bending over people checking their spine and nervous system.

Whatever it is, these small stressors build up hour after hour, day after day, year after year, often to be a worse physical stress than the big ones that we tend to think about. Over time they can lead to significant dysfunction, a loss of health and sometimes even pain.

So how can we prevent these repetitive stressors? Well, variety really is the spice of life. Try not to do the one thing in the one way for too long. If you sit a lot at work, try to get up and move around. If you have a more manual job, try to rotate your role with your colleagues. If you regularly use a computer, you might want to use your left hand on the mouse for a while. Of course well-rounded exercise and stretching will also help add variety of movement to your day.

Remember that some of these repetitive micro-traumas will be unavoidable, so consulting your health care professional about a preventative approach to managing your body rather than waiting for the symptoms is always a good idea.

The Challenge: In the next 21 days identify and remove or limit one of your most chronic repetitive micro-traumas (i.e. assess your work desk and change the ergonomics).

57. Start crawling

Are you aware of the importance of crawling to your child's (or grandchild's) health?

As parents we always want kids to do their best. We want them to learn, to develop, to progress to the next stage. But is this always a good thing? When it comes to crawling, it may not be.

Many parents are unaware of the vital importance of this stage of their child's development. Crawling is in fact vitally important for a baby's neurological development. In particular it helps children to develop good communication between the left and ride sides of their brain. This is due to the 'cross crawl' nature of their movement. A child's crawl should involve using the right arm at the same time as the left leg and vice versa. These left and right brain connections are vital for the body to function at its best and in particular are important for learning.

Crawling also helps your child develop its musculature ready for walking. Combined with regular tummy time in the pre-crawling stage, crawling helps to develop adequate musculature and hence good posture in their neck. Crawling also helps children develop their back extensor muscles ready for proper upright gait.

So whilst it is tempting to want to help your child accelerate past the crawling to the walking phase, it is important to exercise patience. Refrain from using apparatus like baby walkers that tend to encourage your child to start the walking phase before their body is ready, and let your baby develop at her natural rate. Because in the end when it comes to neurological development, posture and learning ability, a slight delay in your baby's progress now may help to prevent a significant developmental delay later in life.

Crawling need not be just for babies either. It is actually an excellent functional exercise for adults (if you aren't afraid to look a little silly).

And remember that if you are still concerned about the time it is taking your baby to progress from crawling to walking, or if your baby is not developing a proper 'cross crawl' crawling pattern, then there may be some developmental or neurological reason. A check-up with a chiropractor or your health care professional may help to alleviate you concerns.

The Challenge: Give your child the chance to learn to crawl and walk in its own time. Resist the urge to rush the transition.

58. Meditate

In his best-selling book *A New Earth*, Eckhart Tolle talks about the importance of breath, amongst many other things. One sentence jumped out at me: he said, "Even if you meditate on your breathing for two hours or more, which some people do, one breath is all you ever need to be aware of – indeed ever can be aware of".

It got me thinking about meditation. I have tried meditation before and struggled with it. So I decided that perhaps I was making it too hard on myself. I decided to try it for a minute and see what happened. It may not be as good as two hours, but it might just make a difference.

Amazingly doing this simple exercise for just one minute is enough to reduce my stress levels significantly when things are flat out. If done regularly it also seems to give me more energy, help me think more clearly and also be more productive throughout the day.

The other thing Eckhart Tolle spoke about (and it seems obvious now) is that I didn't have to consciously breathe. I had previously made the mistake of taking big, slow, conscious breaths and really focusing on how I was breathing. What *A New Earth* points out is, "breathing isn't really something that you do, but something that you witness as it happens". I suddenly realised that rather than consciously breathing, I had to just let my body do what it does naturally: breathe freely and easily and just be present with what happens when it does it.

Now I know some of you might think that meditation is a bit out there for you, but really, this is just a simple breathing exercise. And after all, there is nothing more important to your body than breathing! So give it a go – at the very worst all you will lose is one minute… and who knows what you might gain.

The Challenge: For the next 21 days meditate for one extra minute a day. Repeat this challenge as many times as it takes until you are doing sufficient meditation to create peace in your daily life.

59. Breast feed

I was simply amazed to read the other day that so many people in our society have a problem with breast feeding in public. Given all that we now know about the benefits of breast feeding and the fantastic advantages it provides for both mum and baby, why would anyone have an issue with this?

It is well-recognised that Australian breast feeding rates are lower than they should be. In countries like Norway over 90per cent of mothers are still breast feeding at three months of age. In Australia, that figure is only 64per cent, although most experts recommend that breast feeding to at least one year is ideal. Some of Norway's success comes down to community support like paid maternity leave but it is also due to better acceptance of breast feeding in public. Women aren't made to feel ashamed that they are feeding their babies.

A discreetly breast feeding mother is going to be showing less skin than half of the skimpy bikinis we will see on our beaches this summer, and certainly less than the bare breasts that will be on Bondi beach in Sydney. I don't hear anyone campaigning for more modest bikinis!

Breast feeding has been linked to increased resistance to infectious disease, enhanced immune system function, improved nutrition, reduced obesity, reduced risk of chronic diseases, improved cognitive function and even better health for mum too.

Are we really so out of touch with our natural world that a mother feeding her baby in the most organic, healthy way is an affront to our senses?

So give mums a break. A mother modestly breast feeding in your local cafe is doing you a favour. They are reducing the burden on our overloaded health care system and saving you money!

The Challenge: Create an environment that encourages breastfeeding (be it at work, at home or on the bus) and if you are a breastfeeding Mum, keep up the good work!

60. Focus on normal not common

I read a recent survey suggesting that more than half of the overweight population wrongly believe they are a healthy weight and it got me thinking. How often do we confuse what is common with what is 'normal'.

You only need to look around to see what has become common in our society. It is becoming more and more common to be overweight. It is becoming quite common to have a poor diet. It is becoming very common for people to not exercise enough and even more common for people to be over stressed.

The other common theme running through our society is chronic illness. Strokes, heart attacks, diabetes, cancers and even back pain are all becoming increasingly common ailments. It is becoming so common that people are starting to think it is 'normal'. Well it just isn't true.

The only common thing about all of these chronic illnesses is their cause. These are all 'lifestyle' diseases. They are not caused by germs. They are rarely caused by genes (our genes have changed very little over the last 100,000 years yet these diseases are skyrocketing) and they are not caused by bad luck. They are caused by what you do.

So what is 'normal'? Well 'normal' is a long, happy, healthy life full of energy and vitality. Short of a significant event like a traumatic accident or a genuine genetic disorder there is no reason why you can't have a life like this too.

So stop blaming all your woes on bad luck, bad germs and bad genes and start taking charge of your health. Get out and exercise, start making changes to your diet and start managing your stress levels and you too can have a long, happy, healthy life full of energy and vitality. Your life is what you make it.

The Challenge: For the next 21 days have a good hard look at your health and your lifestyle and start differentiating what is common from what is normal.

61. Cook at home

We all know that so much of our food is over-processed these days. Whether it be the chemicals in the farming, the additives and preservatives and even the containers it is kept in, our food now contains all sorts of nasties. And I use the term 'food' loosely because some of what we eat now has very little nutritional value at all.

But sometimes all it takes to make a significant improvement in your diet is to get back to basics. There is a fantastic book that I have in my library called *Changing Habits, Changing Lives* by Cyndi O'Meara that talks about exactly this. Put simply, if you want it done right when it comes to your food, then it pays to do it yourself.

I know it takes time and effort to prepare a meal yourself but it's probably less than you think. You might even find you enjoy it – and the health benefits are well and truly worth it. The best part is that if you use fresh organic ingredients, you can avoid many of the nasties.

I never cease to be amazed at the quantities of salt and sugar in many of our pre-prepared and take away foods. Even if you make the exact same meal at home, I can guarantee you will use less salt and sugar if you cook it from scratch. Obviously the preservatives and additives are greatly reduced if not eliminated when you make it fresh yourself.

So I know it is old fashioned, but why not start cooking more meals at home? In fact don't just cook at home, cook at home using fresh ingredients and cook the meal from scratch.

The Challenge: For the next 7 weeks cook one extra meal a week at home. Repeat this challenge as many times as it takes until you are preparing most if not all of your weekly meals yourself.

62. Do power training

When most people think about power training, they think of massive over-inflated body builders glistening with fake tan shaping up in front of a mirror. However power training is about a lot more than that, and is important for people of all ages.

One thing people often get confused about is the difference between power and strength. Strength is the amount of force you can produce (i.e. how much weight can you lift) whereas power includes the element of speed (i.e. how fast can you lift/push/pull it).

Of course power is really important in terms of athletic performance but it is really important in terms of injury prevention and everyday wellness as well. The sorts of movements that regularly cause injury are often fast unexpected movements (like catching yourself when you fall). This sort of scenario requires a quick and powerful response from your muscles, and if you don't have sufficient power, will result in injury. By doing power training, you help prepare your muscles for just such a scenario.

Power training is really important for general wellness. It enables you to do resistance exercise and build up your cardio-vascular base at the same time by lifting weights repeatedly and quickly. This enables you to build up your endurance base without losing muscle mass.

"But I don't want to be a body builder", you say. "Is muscle mass really that important?"

Well as it turns out, yes. Muscle tissue is important for your health, not just your looks. It helps you maintain your weight (muscle tissue burns as much as 15 times as many calories as fat tissue does, even at rest) and the American Heart Association has now gone away from the standard half hour cardio a day to recommend strength training at least twice a week to maintain the health of your heart.

So rather than just plodding along doing your resistance exercise at a leisurely pace, why not add some speed to it? Increase your power and you will increase your health.

The Challenge: For the next 7 weeks increase the element of speed to your resistance exercise routine one extra time a week. Repeat this challenge as many times as it takes until you are doing some power training a couple of times as week.

63. Improve your agility

Agility is one of those key fitness skills that is often overlooked. So often we will trundle through our workouts or do repetitive activities that require no change in direction – but how often is the exercise in our daily lives really like that?

Agility is the ability to rapidly change direction without the loss of speed, balance, or body control. It is the ability to use your strength, your endurance, your balance and your coordination in a real-life situation.

Now of course it is easy to see why agility might be important for a footballer or a dancer – it can help them escape an opponent or perform an impossible jump – but it is easy to forget that agility is just as important in everyday life. So often in life things won't happen slowly and they won't happen as we expect them to. When something falls off a ladder above your head, or a car comes screeching around a corner unexpectedly, it is really important that we can move fast but also in a balanced and coordinated way. If we cannot, then we are likely to either get hit by the object or get injured trying to get out of the way.

Agility is really the one skill that enables you to put all of the eight other general fitness skills together into one swift efficient movement.

So how do you train to be more agile?

Well, you train your agility by doing exercise that involves speed, strength, coordination and balance all at the same time. A great example is one of those agility ladders that we see footballers running, hopping and stepping through. They require short, fast movements of the feet in a balanced and coordinated way. Similarly, an agility ball is a great exercise. It is basically a misshaped ball that bounces off of a wall in an unpre-dictable manner (a cricketer's slips cradle is another great example of this). This has the added advantage of adding a degree of unpredictability which adds to the amount of agility required.

So remember, agility is not just for elite athletes. We can all benefit from the ability to move in a fast, coordinated and balanced way when the need arises.

The Challenge: Once a week for the next 7 weeks add some agility to your exercise routine.

64. Add exercise to your daily routine

Many people look at the requirements for 'how much exercise people need in a day to remain healthy', and decide it all seems a bit much: 'Where am I going to find the time to do all that?'

Well the good news is that you don't always have to set aside specific time to exercise. In fact much of your exercise requirement can be taken up whilst you are at work, while you are doing the shopping and even when you are catching up with friends. The key is to incorporate your exercise into your activities of daily living (ADL).

For example, rather than driving round and round at the supermarket looking for that perfect park near the entrance, why not take that space at the very back of the car park? You will save yourself time and stress and you will get a nice little walk to the shops to boot. There's five minutes each way of walking!

The old cliché at work is to take the stairs rather than the lift, but it really does work (assuming you have a multi-story workplace). This simple exercise can easily add 20 minutes of exercise into every day as you head into work, out for a meeting, out for lunch and then home again. If your office doesn't have stairs, you may consider parking a little way away or getting public transport, and then walking in to get the same effect. There's another 20 minutes each day!

And instead of catching up with your friends at the coffee shop for a chin wag, why not meet them at the oval or the beach and go for a nice talk while you chat away? You can easily slide in 30 minutes of exercise and the best bit is, you will be so busy chatting you won't even notice. There's a bonus 30 mins exercise!

The Challenge: For the next 21 days find one thing you can do to incorporate some exercise into your daily routine.

65. Get enough movement

In our modern lifestyles many of us spend way too much time sitting and don't get anywhere near enough exercise. In fact one of the most common questions I get from people is, 'How much exercise is enough?'

We often hear that we should be doing half an hour of walking a day to keep our heart healthy, but what about the rest of our body? Obviously walking is only one form of exercise and doesn't test our strength, power, balance or coordination. So obviously there is more to it than that. The recommendation to walk is not a bad idea, but like many of these recommendations it is based on the minimum amount of work you can do to reduce the incidence of a particular condition (in this case heart disease). It is not based on how much exercise you need to function at your best or to be 100per cent healthy.

So how do we figure out how much – and what types – of exercise we need? Well, the best way to work it out is to look at how much exercise our bodies are designed to do. I mean think about it: we evolved over millions of years to be hunter-gatherers: walking, running, climbing, throwing, tackling and stretching for hours each day, and even finding time and energy to dance in the evening. So this is what our bodies have evolved to expect, and what they need in order to maintain their homeostasis (health).

If we look at studies estimating what an 80kg Palaeolithic (caveman) male did each day, we find that he burnt around 4000 calories. Around half of those are burned doing normal bodily functions like thinking, digesting and healing, but still that leaves 2000 calories a day that primitive man burnt by doing physical activity. Contrast that to a modern 80kg male, who burns just 2720 calories a day – and only 696 of those are from physical activity. In other words, we aren't doing anywhere near enough.

So what does 2000 calories a day of physical activity equate to? Well, it would be two hours of jogging, four hours of walking, three hours of weight training, two hours of sprinting, or 3.5 hours of dancing.

I know, I know, it's a lot, isn't it! The good news is that you don't need to do all that. If you are eating the right stuff you are going to have to work very, very hard to eat 4000 calories, and if you are smart about it, you can burn over half of those calories doing regular daily activities like walking to work or taking the stairs.

So what's left? Well, each day you should be aiming to do 30-60 minutes of exercise. This should include endurance exercise, balance and accuracy training each day, and two to three times a week some strength, power, stamina, coordination and agility training. Sounds like a lot, but remember you don't have to do all of these skills separately. In fact a well designed half-hour workout might contain all of these key elements.

And please don't fall for the trap of saying that you are too tired or you don't have enough time to do this exercise. I can guarantee you that if you just do it, you will get more energy than you can imagine and your increased productivity will means that it actually frees up more time in your day.

So if you don't do any fitness now don't try and do all of this tomorrow. Take it easy, pick one small step that you can start doing tomorrow and gradually build it from there and you WILL reap the rewards.

The Challenge: For the next 7 weeks add an extra half an hour of exercise each week. Repeat this challenge as many times as it takes until you are doing 30-60 minutes of exercise a day.

66. Use affirmations

Everybody knows someone who is painfully positive. No matter what is going on in their lives they still approach it with childlike enthusiasm and a huge smile on their face. We also all know that person who is the exact opposite. They could win the top prize in the weekday lotto and complain that it didn't pay very well. In fact of you put these two people into exactly the same situation (stimulus) they would react very differently to each other, how is this possible? Aren't we all wired the same?

The answer may come down to a thought addiction.

Now I know what you're thinking, don't be ridiculous. How could you possibly be addicted to a thought!

Well as it turns out it is exactly the same as any other addiction. When you have a thought (be it positive or negative) it fires off certain pathways in your brain. If over time you continually fire the same pathway it will become sensitized. This means that more neurons form along this pathway and it also fires off easier, hence making it easier to have these thoughts again in the future.

Because these pathways are being continually fired we also become addicted to the chemicals being released in our brain. This means that not only are these thoughts more easily entertained, we also actively seek them to feed our addiction, just like a smoker seeks nicotine to set off the nicotinic receptors in the brain.

The good news is we can choose which thoughts we are addicted to.

You can sensitise positive pathways by using positive self-talk, affirmations and by focusing on what you have achieved. This sets off and sensitises the pathways in your brain that release of dopamine and serotonin (the feel good chemicals). Not only do these chemicals make you feel better, they also switch off the stress response in your body which has been linked to many chronic diseases, including strokes, cancers, diabetes and heart attacks.

Conversely when you think negative thoughts, bitch about others or let fear rule your life you are feeding your negative thought addiction and setting yourself up for a life of negativity, fear and poor health.

Remember that you are still being "real" and you are still recognising the "truth" of the situation and you are still dealing with it. It is just that now you are consciously choosing how you want to perceive that situation and reacting to it in a much more positive (and useful) fashion.

The Challenge: Create a positive affirmation. Write it in the first person and in present tense (I am/I do) and make sure it is positive (I do, NOT I won't). Read it out once a day for the next 21 days with purpose.

67. Utilise mentors and mates

When you are trying to make healthy lifestyle change one of the hardest things can be the lack of support or even open ridicule of those around you. People can be quite confronted by your choices, as if you were making a personal attack on the lifestyle they are accustomed to. So choosing to surround yourself with people who support your choices can be very important to your journey.

I have been very fortunate that throughout the years I have had a large number of fantastic mentors to help me along the way. Some of these have been practitioners I have seen, some have been seminars I have been to, some have been wonderful books or websites I have read and others have been just good mates who are on a similar journey. Whatever the source, I have learnt a lot. In fact pretty much everything you have read in my columns, on my website or even in this book has been begged, borrowed or stolen from one of these mentors.

So who are you surrounding yourself with? Are they helping or hindering your journey?

Now I am not by any means saying ditch all your old friends, but you may need to complement them with a few more positive mentors. What should you look for in a good mentor? Well, there are several factors. They need to have more knowledge than you. They need to have more passion and/or discipline than you. They need to be further along their journey than you. They need to be a better problem-solver than you to help tailor your wellness changes. They would also need to be able to help you set achievable goals and action steps.

Sounds like an impossible person to find, doesn't it? Well the good news is that these don't all need to be one person. There may be different people or even books or websites that help to mentor you in each of these areas. In fact you may even have different people for different aspects of your health and wellness. The person you turn to for dietary advice may be very different to the person who helps you think more positively. And the person who helps you learn what a good diet is may not be the best person to motivate you to do it, or plan your meals.

So start finding yourself some wellness mentors. Don't worry, they are all around you if you look, and they will make your journey to wellness much easier! In fact why not encourage a mate to get this book too so that you can go through the journey together and keep each other accountable?

The challenge: In the next 21 days find one mentor or mate who can help you on your wellness journey and make a plan to catch up regularly. This may mean a catch up for a cup of tea, an appointment with a practitioner or even just a regular time when you read an inspiring book.

68. Have a healthy scepticism

Scepticism can be defined as a studied attitude of questioning and doubt. A healthy degree of scepticism is an important tool to have in all aspects of your life and health is no exception. It used to be that a man in a white coat would tell us what we needed to do and we would just blindly follow the leader, but not anymore. Now we have access to a wealth of information from a wide variety of sources – some reliable, some not so much – and it is up to each of us to find what works for you. It also used to be the case that we could trust the media (to a reasonable extent) to report the facts. Now it seems that we are more concerned with a good story than a truthful one.

Recently I have come across a number of people who define themselves as sceptics. When I investigated further, though, these people weren't being sceptical at all. They were rigidly defending one side of an argument by only looking at one side of the facts, most often the status quo.

So how can you exercise a healthy degree of scepticism when it comes to healthcare?

Actively search for information. This is perhaps the easiest thing to do with all of our modern technology, but perhaps also the hardest thing to do well – there is such a wealth of information out there!

Get your info from more than one source. If you want to show a healthy scepticism, it is really important that you know the whole story. Otherwise it would be a bit like voting based purely on the voting card of one political party – despite their obvious political nous and intelligence, you will not get the whole story.

Give all health care the same degree of scepticism. Some people will often be highly sceptical of what they consider to be alternative healthcare, but do you critique all of the information presented to you in the same fashion?

Understand the limitations of research. Research is only as good as the questions that are asked. When researchers asked 'Is Vioxx good for arthritis?', the answer was yes. However when they altered the question later on (after many deaths) to, 'Is Vioxx good for you?', the answer came back a resounding NO. Research is also only as good as the integrity and independence of the researchers. Often research will not be independently funded and there is no requirement to publish all of the research (you can do 10 studies, only one of which has a favourable result, and then only publish the favourable one). Research is also dependent on the amount of funding available. It can cost a lot of time and money to do high quality research... meaning that sometimes the best research is done where the most money can be made, not where the best results can be found. Don't get me wrong, research is very important, but it too needs to be read with a healthy dose of scepticism.

Take charge of your health. Remember that the only person in charge of your health is you. You are the one who ultimately makes every decision about your healthcare and therefore your health outcomes. Make all of your choices with a healthy degree of scepticism and you will go a long way to finding good health.

So start looking at everything you do in your life that affects your health and ask yourself why you do it. Is it just habit? Is it just following the crowd? Or is it that you have thoroughly researched both sides of the equation and consciously decided for yourself what is right for you.

The challenge: In the next 21 days find one thing that you do in your life that affects your health (whether it is something you consider healthy or not) and look at it sceptically. It might be your breakfast, or what you drink or even what you say to yourself. Does it stack up?

69. Defeat fear

Fear is the guiding emotion for so many people in our society and it is terrible for your health. Not only is fear a negative thought that stimulates the release of stress hormones in your body, it can also adversely affect your health choices.

Fear tends us towards reactive health choices, and towards doing what everyone else is doing. It causes us to avoid standing out from the crowd.

'I don't want to stand out', you say?

Well the problem is that the crowd is incredibly unhealthy. As many as 80per cent of society is suffering from chronic disease, over a half of us are overweight, and almost a quarter take pain relievers on a daily basis. So, do you really want to blend in with the crowd?

Wellness involves making health choices based around what you want to do, or what you would love to do, rather than around what you don't want to do, or what you are scared of. It also involves courage. After all, we don't ever really know 100per cent whether a health change is going to be good for us or not. If I start running more I might get fitter and healthier, or I might get an injury – and the research around what is healthy to eat and what is not seems to change on a daily basis.

But if you truly want to get healthy, you need to start making choices based around what you want to do and who you want to be, rather than making decisions out of fear.

So as Susan Jeffers says in her fantastic book of the same title, 'Feel the fear and do it anyway!' and you will start to make decisions based on what you need to do to get healthy rather than what the crowd think you should do.

The challenge: In the next 21 days look at one health decision you have been contemplating and ask yourself, 'What would I do if I didn't care what other people thought or said'.

70. Eat small fish

The humble seafood dinner has become a victim of the pollution of our environment. Not so long ago you could have happily recommended people eat a couple of serves of fish a week, content in the knowledge that it was great for them. After all, fish are a great source of essential fats, in particular Omega 3's which are great for your body in many ways. They are protective for your heart and nourishing for your brain. They are also a great source of protein to give you long-lasting energy and balance out our carbohydrate-laden diets.

So what is the concern?

In a word: mercury. Because of our pollution of the environment, especially from coal-fired power stations and mining, we have seen a dramatic increase in mercury – and particularly in our fish. In fact the contamination of Pacific fish (especially tuna) has increased by a whopping 30per cent since 1990! It is also important to remember that mercury never leaves your body and toxicity can result in paraesthesia, depression, and blurred vision, and can have an even more devastating impact on a developing fetus or an infant including arrhythmias of the heart, headaches and effects on attention span, memory and coordination.

So should we avoid fish all together? Well, at this stage, I would say no. We know that Omega 3's and protein have fantastic health benefits but we don't know what else in fish is beneficial for our health. As is often the case I have no doubt that in future years we will find out that there is something in the whole fish that is more than just the sum of its parts and more than we can get in a capsule.

I recommend eating small fish regularly.

Why small fish? Well in the fish food chain, the small fish get eaten by the medium-sized fish, meaning that the medium-sized fish have not only the mercury they got from their environment but also that from all the small fish they ate. The large fish of course has its own mercury, plus that of the medium fish, plus that of the many small fish... you get the idea. So stay clear of large fish like tuna, flake and swordfish, and instead choose smaller fish like sardines, anchovies and Tommy Roughs. And due to the increased sensitivity of the fetus if you are pregnant it might pay to avoid the fish all together just for the next nine months and go for capsules instead.

And if we keep polluting waterways the way we are, don't be surprised if in a few years time if you hear me reluctantly recommending that you avoid fish all together.

The challenge: For the next 7 weeks eat one extra meal of small fish a week. Repeat this challenge as many times as it takes until you are eating a couple of serves of small fish a week.

71. Eat some whole grains

Whenever I speak to people about the excessive amounts of processed carbs, breads grains and cereals in our modern diets, I invariably get the question, 'What about whole grains? They're good for you, aren't they?' Well, the answer is a little complicated, but worth going through here.

What you need to remember is that until around 5,000 years ago we didn't have the mechanical capabilities to process grains on a large scale. If you wanted to process grain you had to do it by hand, and it was a very labour intensive practice. As such it was a difficult way to get nutrients and to get sustenance, and so it wasn't done very much. As it turns out, this was a good thing. Processed grains and cereals are essentially sugars that are released into our blood stream very quickly. They cause a spike and then a crash in our blood sugar levels, and as a result have been linked to many of our chronic diseases – including, most recently, heart disease according to The Archives of Internal Medicine.

So why are there so many studies showing the benefits of whole grains? Well, quite simply, they are better than more processed varieties. For example, wholegrain bread is much better for you than white bread. So if the majority of the population are eating white bread and you do a study that gets a group of them to eat wholegrain bread, their health would improve. But what about if you did another study where the people ate no bread at all – where in fact they ate only what our hunter-gatherer ancestors ate? Well, then they would be healthier again! You see, it all depends on the question the study asks, and 'healthier' does not equal 'healthiest'.

And not all whole grains are created equal, either. The entire point of a wholegrain should be that is a whole grain (sounds simple doesn't it). But what that means is that it is the whole grain, unprocessed, un-milled: in other words it still looks like a grain. This means that it contains lots of coarse fibre that is good for your digestion, and the sugars get released much slower into your blood stream. If, however, you get that whole grain and mill it to a pulp where it is so fine that you don't even recognise the bread as whole grain, then you are losing most of the benefits.

So eat a small amount of wholegrain in your diet, but make sure that they are actual 'whole grains'. Something like a handful of brown rice in a dish is not going to throw out your sugar metabolism, whereas a slice of highly processed 'wholegrain' bread probably will.

The Challenge: Once a week for the next 7 weeks remove one serve of processed grains or replace one serve with real whole grains. Repeat as many times as you like to a maximum of one small serve of whole grains a day.

72. Drink healthy juice

Juicing seems to be one of those things that people either love or hate in terms of health benefits. On one hand, it is a fantastic way to get a concentrated injection of natural nutrients. Raw whole fruits are a great way to supplement your diet. On the other hand there is more in the fruit than just the water soluble nutrients. Most people don't realise that fruits and vegetables are in fact the best source of fibre. You can also get more pieces of fruit (and in particular sugar) concentrated into a glass of juice than you would ever consume in one session.

So what is the answer?

Well, juice can be a really important part of your diet so long as you consume it intelligently. Here are five great tips to help you continue to enjoy your juice.

1. Make sure that your juices contain mostly vegetables (and a little bit of fruit for sweetness) to help minimise the sugar content.

2. Dilute your juice with water. I usually use around one part juice to four parts water. This ensures you get a nice refreshing drink, an important nutrient top up and not too much of a sugar overload whilst also helping to hydrate your body.

3. Add some protein into your juice. This helps to minimise the sugar rush and provides you with a more sustaining, nourishing, filling drink. Add some ground up nuts or a raw egg to help balance out the sugary juice. Trust me, it tastes better than it sounds! (and if you just can't bear the thought just make sure you eat some protein on the side).

4. Make your own juice using fresh organic fruits and vegetables to avoid the added sugar, sweeteners, flavourings and preservatives that are found in many of

our off-the-shelf juices.

5. Get the majority of your fluids from pure water rather than juice. Unless you are doing huge amounts of exercise, you simply don't need all those extra calories.

More often than not you are better off eating the whole fruits and vegetables than the juice. But if you do it intelligently, you can enjoy a fresh fruit and vegetable (and maybe protein) juice as part of a balanced diet.

The challenge: For the next 21 days replace one soft drink, cordial or sports drink a week with a fruit juice. Or if you already drink fruit juice replace one regular fruit juice with a fruit and vegetable juice. Or replace one regular fruit juice with a fresh squeezed one. Or if you already drink fresh squeezed fruit and vegetable juice drink one a week with some added protein.

73. Healthy eating ratios

We all know that we are becoming a nation, in fact a world, of overweight people. In fact Australia is leading the way with more overweight people than any other developed nation. Many people and even scientists have assumed that it is because we are eating more fats. The facts are, though, we are eating the same amounts of fat we always have, and what we are actually eating much more of is carbohydrates: sugars, breads, grains and cereals.

If you look right back to our hunter-gatherer ancestors, studies show that they ate around 30-45per cent fat, 20-35per cent protein and 25-40per cent carbs. Compare that to our modern diet where we average 35-40per cent fat, 15-20per cent protein and a whopping 45-55per cent carbohydrates. It is clear to see that our per centage fat intakes have not changed much. Of course what has changed is the *types* of fat we eat, but that is for another chapter.

The other thing that is obvious from these stats is that we are eating a lot less protein and a lot more carbohydrates. Hardly surprising given the food choices we have around us. Everywhere you look there are sugary foods, soft drinks, breads, grains and cereals. I mean just check out the food pyramid (created largely by farmers in 1910) if you don't believe me.

This over-reliance on processed carbohydrates is leading to many of the health problems we see around us. Obesity for starters – I mean think about it, how do you fatten up a cow? You feed it lots of grains and cereals! What about diabetes and insulin resistance? That's a product of our excessive sugar consumption. How about our roller coaster energy levels – you know, those mid-morning and mid-afternoon crashes? They're a result of spikes of sugary energy followed by crashes due to the speed at which it is processed by our bodies. I could go on and on.

Now I am not saying that you should eliminate carbohydrates all together, or even that you should eat as little as possible. Healthy carbohydrates (from fruits and particularly vegetables) are important and just like your hunter-gatherer ancestors, they should make up around 25-40per cent of your diet. But for most people this means you should eat less carbs and in particular healthier carbs than you do right now. Similarly, you should look for ways to increase your healthy protein intake. By healthy proteins I mean natural ones. Nuts, eggs, healthy meats, mushrooms etc. are all healthy ways to improve your protein intake.

So start to increase the healthy proteins in your diet and feel the difference in both your health and your energy levels.

The challenge: For the next 7 weeks find one meal a week that is high in carbohydrates and replace it with one that is an equal balance of healthy (natural) fats, proteins and carbohydrates. Think eggs, healthy meats, nuts and seeds and legumes to get the protein and fat content up.

74. Don't shop hungry

The battle to eat healthily is often won and lost at the shops. If you buy healthy stuff during your weekly shop, you are much more likely to be eating healthily throughout the week. I mean let's face it, if you have one of those weak moments when you are home and there is something naughty in the fridge, you are much more likely to eat it then if you had to get dressed, get in the car, drive down to the shops, buy it and drive home again.

One of the best ways to help yourself buy healthy options at the shops is to never shop hungry. When you are hungry you will often crave all of those things you know you shouldn't be eating. You will also find it much harder to resist temptation.

Another great simple step is to make a list and stick to it. It is so easy to be tempted once you are at the shops by all of those tasty treats that are placed in just the right places by behavioural experts with just the right colours and words designed by expert marketers, all designed to make them irresistible to you.

So eat a good meal and create a healthy list, it will make a massive difference to your willpower in the aisles, and an even bigger difference to the goodness of your weekly meals and snacks.

The challenge: For the next 21 days each time you go shopping, eat a nice, healthy, filling (high protein) snack before heading out to the shops. Then make a list at home away from all of those temptations and decide to stick to it.

75. Create a vision board

One of the best ways to ensure that you are focused and on purpose is to create a vision board. Put simply it's a visual representation of your goals and dreams. It is one thing to have a written statement of purpose and written goals but for many people (myself included) putting it into a picture form makes it more real, more tangible somehow and can be really inspiring.

To do this first you need to figure out what you want in life (your goals and dreams) so if you haven't done your statement of purpose (chapter one) that is probably the best place to start. Once you have defined your statement of purpose, what you really want you can start to think about the trappings that go along with that.

It might be material things like a flash car, a fancy wardrobe or a beautiful house. It might be more immaterial things like a great relationship, a family or a great group of friends, it might be a business goal like your very own shop you always dreamed of, it might be a financial thing like a certain amount of money or a certain income, or it might be a health goal like a fit body, a certain weight or an attractive set of legs.

Put simply, you need to figure out all the things you really want in life – be they relationships, family, money, health, fitness, cars, jobs, whatever it is – and create a picture board with all of these things on it. If you aren't really into computers (or you just like doing it this way) you can go around collecting pictures from magazines, newspapers, adverts and all over the place (be sure to ask for permission first) or in this digital world it can be even easier. I like to just search in Google images on the computer. I enter in the appropriate search word, troll through until I find the image I want and then cut and paste it into a document (say a PowerPoint page). That way I can arrange all of the pictures on the one page and I can add text if I like to make it more clear. I also add my statement of purpose at the bottom to put the goals into context because remember I only want to get these things if I can do it in a way that fits with my statement of purpose (I don't want the flash car if I have to steal it or earn it in a way that doesn't benefit others).

So create a vision board and stick it up somewhere you will see it every day. You will be amazed at how it starts to guide your mind to search for opportunities to achieve the very things that you want most in life.

The challenge: In the next 21 days create a vision board and put it somewhere you will see it every day.

76. Get a good sleep

Are you one of the 75 per cent of adults who frequently suffer from sleep problems?

Poor sleep can lead to:

- Poor health
- Low productivity at work
- Danger on the roads (less alert)
- Impaired memory
- Fertility problems
- Social and intimate relationship problems

And it's not just the quantity of sleep that is important, but the quality as well. Only 50 per cent of people report that they sleep well on most nights and 1 in 4 people say sleep problems have some influence on their daily lives.

And just because you are not noticing any symptoms does not mean that you are in the clear. Without a doubt, sleeping well is absolutely essential if you are ever to achieve optimal health and wellness, so even if you are feeling fine, your lack of quality sleep is affecting your body's performance.

Getting enough sleep is also vitally important to your work performance. It will affect almost everything from your ability to think clearly and problem-solve, to your productivity and even your work relationships.

Many animals realise that a great way to combat lack of sleep is the midday nap, in fact my (not so little) puppy is demonstrating it right now. Research on napping suggests that an afternoon nap as short as 10 minutes can enhance alertness, mood, and mental performance, especially after a night of poor sleep. In fact it seems that a nap shorter than 10 minutes has no desirable effect and that anything longer than half an hour leads to you feeling even drowsier in the afternoon.

Here are a few key tips I give my clients to help them sleep better.

1. Avoid alcohol and caffeine, especially in the evening
2. Late evening/bedtime snacks (particularly grains and sugars) will inhibit your sleep.
3. Wind down before you go to bed: relax and meditate, or read a book.
4. Sleep in complete darkness or as close to it as possible. If there is even the tiniest bit of light in the room it can disrupt your circadian rhythm and your pineal gland's production of melatonin and serotonin.
5. Ensure that you are getting quality and quantity of spinal movement during the day. This means good quality exercise and perhaps a visit to your local chiropractor. This helps switch off the stress response in your body and allows you to fully relax.
6. Try a midday nap to help you perform better in the afternoon.

The challenge: For the next 7 weeks set aside one day a week where you follow at least the first five of these rules. Repeat this challenge as many times as it takes until you are doing this 6-7 nights a week.

77. Focus on what you can control

How much of our energy in our daily life do we spend worrying about things that we can't control? All sorts of things, from a car crash on the news, to the way that someone else feels about us, to the next global recession. We worry about things that were done in the past and things that might happen in the future. We worry and worry and worry and it is making us sick.

The stress response in your body is a powerful thing. It is linked to strokes, cancers, heart disease and diabetes, and every time we worry, we switch it on. In fact if we constantly worry, it probably never switches off.

So what is the answer to all this worrying?

It is called present time consciousness. Essentially it means focusing on the job at hand. Now that doesn't mean you can't learn from past mistakes, and it doesn't mean that you can't plan for the future. What it does mean, though, is that you only focus on the past events and future hypotheticals that directly relate to the job at hand right now. You focus on the things that you can control, the things that you can influence to help make the situation better. After all, if it is not within your sphere of influence, then you are not doing anyone any good by worrying about it. You are not helping solve the problem and you are not helping your own health and wellbeing.

One of the best ways to reduce the amount you are worrying is to stop watching as much mainstream media. Our TVs, radios and newspapers are becoming more and more negative and sensationalist in their content. In fact you are much more likely to see a negative story from the other side of the world than you are to see a positive story from your very own backyard. Taking in too much mainstream media is a great way to set your mind off worrying about something you have no influence over.

So start focusing on the present and stop worrying about

things you can't control. After all, you are always better off working for a solution than worrying about a problem.

The challenge: Set aside one whole day where you notice what you are worrying about and write them down. Then analyse these things to see whether they were within your sphere of influence and for the next 21 days choose to release the ones that are not. Repeat this challenge as many times as it takes until you are regularly practicing present time consciousness.

78. Good time management

You don't need me to tell you that our lives are becoming busier and busier and that time pressures are one of the biggest stressors we have. Often the biggest challenge is not how much time we actually have but how effectively we are using it. Our modern lives are so full of distractions and time wasters that we often spend all our time and energy doing stuff that doesn't really matter.

Your daily tasks can be broken down into four categories: important stuff that is urgent, important stuff that is not urgent, unimportant stuff that is urgent, and unimportant stuff that is not urgent.

Usually the important, urgent stuff is the first thing that gets ticked off from our list. It is a no brainer, it needs to be done and it needs to be done NOW so we do it, no questions asked. So far, so good.

Unfortunately for most people, the second item on their list is the urgent unimportant stuff. It is easy to push those long-term important tasks into the background because there are emails in your Inbox, a great show on TV right now, or a great piece of gossip to share. The problem with this is that the non-urgent important stuff gets shoved out the way and often, in fact, never gets done. These are also the things that stress us out. Hour after hour, day after day, we keep saying to ourselves 'gee, I really need to get that done', or 'when am I ever going to find time to live that dream?'

The key to getting these big long-term goals achieved is to prioritise your actions. Take a look at your mission statement (chapter 1) and analyse your daily activities with that vision in mind. Which of these tasks are really helping you achieve what you want to achieve in life, and which are just wasting your time? In fact the best way to do this is to number them in order, from most important to least. Then when you sit down to plan your day, or are trying to figure out what to do next, have a look at your priorities list. Prioritise those important ones first and you will find you are not only getting more done with your time, but you will be less stressed as well.

The challenge: Get out a piece of paper and divide it up into 4 quadrants, labelled important/urgent, unimportant/urgent, important/non-urgent and unimportant/non-urgent. Now think of everything you have to do today (or tomorrow if it is evening) and place them all in one of these 4 quadrants. Now number them in order of importance. Repeat this challenge as many times as it takes until you get in the habit of prioritising your important/non-urgent tasks appropriately.

79. Grow your own food

I was just reading in a magazine the other day that the latest "trend' is veggie patches and I was very pleased. The humble vegetable patch is good for your health in so many ways:

1. If you are growing lots of vegetables, chances are you are eating lots of vegetables and we all know that they are great for your health.
2. Home-grown food tastes fantastic so you will be even more likely to eat more fruits and veggies.
3. You have the opportunity to grow organic. Since you control the entire process you can determine what does and does not end up in your food.
4. You have an excuse to get outside and do some exercise.
5. Gardening is a great way to relax and unwind.
6. Vegetable patches are a great opportunity to teach your kids about what real food is and where it comes from. If you can teach your kids to appreciate real, fresh, home-grown and cooked food from a young age, it will stay with them for life.
7. Patience and discipline. Both of these life skills are essential if you want to grow great vegetables. Regular watering, feeding and plant care are essential to get a good crop and you will need to keep it up long enough to harvest.
8. It is a great analogy for your health. Just as you need to weed, fertilise and cultivate your veggie patch so you need to look after your body.

The challenge: In the next 21 days get out in the garden and create an organic vegetable patch. Even if you only have time or space for a pot plant start with some lovely fresh herbs. Or if you already have a vegetable patch that isn't organic find an alternative to the chemicals and sprays.

80. Make your own baby food

Introducing solids is a very important step in your child's development and often parents will put a lot more thought into what they feed their babies than what they feed themselves. However I am constantly surprised at the amounts of processed foods, chemical additives, pesticides and processed carbohydrates that I constantly see babies being fed. And I am even more blown away by how many people think it is remarkable enough to stop me in the street and comment that my 18 month old son is eating an apple, or a bunch of grapes, surely a sign of the times.

Even fruits and vegetables like apples, pears, celery and spinach can be surprisingly high in pesticides. Whilst these pesticides and sprays have been declared to be safe at lower levels in isolation, we really have no knowledge of the compounding effect of these small amounts in many different foods, particularly on a developing baby.

Many of the commercially available baby foods contain many other additives and chemicals including preservatives and flavourings that your baby simply doesn't need. They also contain ingredients that you probably wouldn't put into your baby's food if you were to make it yourself including sugars, salt and fat. Plus, they are often cooked at high temperatures in order to kill bacteria – unfortunately this heat treatment often destroys vital vitamins and minerals as well.

The other thing that troubles me in babies' food is the reliance on breads, grains and cereals, including the oft-loved baby rusks. It is tempting to feed your baby large quantities of these foods due to the fact they are easy to make, easy to transport and often easy to get the baby to eat. However the high sugar (carbohydrate) content of these foods and the pace at which these sugars are released into the bloodstream due to the highly processed nature is not ideal. Firstly, it means that your baby is not getting a sustained energy release. The quick release of these sugars tends to give your baby a quick release of energy followed by a crash later on (thus a tired, grumpy baby). Secondly, consuming this sugar intake as a baby can affect the ability to process sugars later on. As a result of this we are seeing increased cases of insulin resistance from a younger and younger age, leading to a greater chance of diabetes and other illnesses later on in life.

And don't forget to think about the containers you are putting your baby food into. Many of the plastic containers contain BPA, which has been shown to be harmful for your baby's health (see chapter 91).

The challenge: For the next 7 weeks replace one of your baby's meals a week with homemade food from healthy meats, fruits, vegetables, nuts (assuming no allergy) and seeds. Repeat this challenge as many times as it takes until your baby is eating only fresh healthy ingredients.

81. Get into nature.

Getting out into nature is good for your health. I don't have any gold standard, double-blind, randomised control studies to prove it, but I innately know it to be true – and there are very sound reasons as to why.

Firstly, spending time in nature incorporates exercise. In almost every instance, getting out into nature involves walking, running, climbing or paddling your way around, and I don't think I need to spend too much time here explaining to you just how good that is.

Secondly, it involves fresh air. You only need to go for a stroll around the inner city for 10 minutes to realise that the quality of the air we breathe isn't what it used to be. The more we can get out into nature, get some fresh air into our lungs and reduce the chemical (pollution) load on our lungs, the better we will be.

Thirdly it involves de-stressing. There is just something about nature that is great for reducing stress. The exercise plays a significant role, as does the fresh air and the quiet thinking time. Whatever it is, though, there is no doubt that getting into nature will leave you feeling less stressed, and given the links between stress and chronic disease, this will have an impact on your health.

Fourthly, it involves getting in touch with nature. This is one of those intangible benefits, but there is no doubt that getting into nature and seeing the beautiful balance of a natural, undisturbed ecosystem at work gives us pause to think about our own bodies and what kind of ecosystem we are maintaining. We understand that a forest needs nutrients (minerals, sunlight, water) and we understand that it needs no toxicity (pollution, woodchoppers, chemical sprays), and so it causes us to think (consciously or subconsciously) about the kinds of nutrients and toxicities we are creating around our own body.

The challenge: Set aside a time in the next 21 days to spend some time out in nature. Repeat this challenge as many times as it takes until spending a little time in nature is a regular habit.

82. Invest time

I read a great quote from Dr John Demartini today: "If you don't fill your day with high priorities, it will automatically be filled with low priorities." How often have you wanted to make a change that you knew would be beneficial to your health but didn't have the time? We all know that there are positive steps we could start tomorrow that would have a real, tangible effect on our health and our life.

There are 24 hours in a day, seven days a week and the average life span is in the seventies so in reality most of the time it comes down to what you are prioritising, not really how much time you actually have. Whenever surveys are done about what people value the most, health invariably comes in very high, if not at the top of the list. Yet if you were to do another survey measuring what people actually spend their time doing, it wouldn't be high at all.

If you are adamant that you just don't have any time at all, I want you to do one thing for me. Firstly write a list of your priorities – the things that are most important to you in life – friends, family, health, money etc. (Check these against your mission statement to see if they fit). This is your 'To Do' list. For the next week, keep a very strict diary. Write down everything you are doing and how much time you are spending doing it, including time watching TV, time on the Internet, time gossiping, time procrastinating, time worrying etc. This is your 'Do' list. You will be amazed (and maybe a little embarrassed) at just how much time you spend doing these things. Now go back and look at your list of priorities and see how much time you are spending on your top five.

You will soon realise that there is time available, but you are not prioritising correctly. So start consciously filling your day with high priorities first. And if health is one of your high priorities, then start allocating time to get healthy. You're worth it!

The challenge: Create a 'Do' and a 'To Do' list. For the next 21 days find one thing on 'Do' list that you can handle not doing and reduce the time you're doing it. Now use that time to do the one thing on your 'To Do' list that you would most like to be doing. Repeat this as many times as it takes until you are comfortable with how you are achieving your priorities.

83. Use healthy oils and fats

Did you know that the latest research shows that it is the type of fat that you eat and not the total amount of fat you eat that has the greatest impact on your weight and your health?

In fact if you look back at what our ancestors ate, studies have shown that the typical hunter gatherer's diet was 30-45per cent fat, whilst the typical Western diet contains 35-40per cent fat – pretty much exactly the same. What has changed markedly along with our waistlines is the type of fat we eat (as well as the protein-to-carbohydrate ratios and exercise levels).

Previously our diets were rich in healthy fats. The sort of fats that we get from fish, grass-fed, free range meats and flaxseed oil are very different from the fat in your average hamburger.

Studies have shown that populations like the people of Crete and the Inuits of Greenland and Denmark had relatively high fat intakes, yet low incidences of heart disease and cancer.

Another study by the USDA in 1995 showed that so long as people ate healthy ratios of fat they had the same changes in total and LDL cholesterol whether their diet was 22per cent or 39per cent fat. In other words, it wasn't a reduction in the amount of fat that altered their cholesterol profile; it was a change in the ratios of different fats (i.e. more healthy omega 3 laden fats). The changes to our fat intake don't end there. It is not just the reduction in healthy fats that is damaging our health; it is the increased intake of unhealthy fats. One of the biggest culprits here is trans-fats. These fats are found in virtually all processed foods, sometimes labelled as trans-fats but more often hidden as hydrogenated or partially hydrogenated fats. These fats not only adversely affect your cholesterol profile but are linked to many other lifestyle diseases.

So remember, whether you are trying to lose weight or just be as healthy as you can be, fat is not the enemy. In fact healthy natural fats from fish, grass-fed meats, flaxseed oil, coconut and olive oil (amongst others) are an essential part of any healthy diet.

The Challenge: For the next 21 days replace one unhealthy (unnatural) fat in your diet with a healthy (natural) one. Repeat this challenge as many times as it takes until your diet consists as close as possible to entirely healthy fats.

84. Be informed

People often ask me if it is 'worth' going to see their doctor or 'worth' going to see a podiatrist or 'worth' going and seeing a naturopath about a specific condition or problem. They are often surprised when my answer invariably comes back as a yes. People tend to think that because I'm a wellness expert and columnist, I have all the answers and that I wouldn't want to them to go and get a second opinion that may differ from mine.

In reality nothing could be further from the truth. Wellness is all about finding out as much information as possible about a problem and about its possible solutions, so that you can take charge of your health care decisions and make an informed choice. Gone are the days when people just went into their trusted doctor and blindly took whatever pill or potion they were given, and rightly so.

We have seen that many of those blindly followed recommendations have led to less than ideal, sometimes even disastrous consequences, and so we now expect more. So not only do we need to seek as many opinions as possible on what to do and how to do it, we also need to be prepared to take that information, compare it, digest it and make our own decision about the best course of action for us.

When I am confronted with a health question or am doing some research I will always try and look at the problem from as many different angles as possible. I will research what the medical solution to it is, I will look at what the alternatives are and then I will look at what tools the body already has to deal with such issues, and I will come up with the best course of action for me or my family – which is then the course of action I recommend to my clients and readers. Usually I will come up with the same answer I had to start with, and usually for me it will revolve around eating well, thinking well, moving well and getting regular chiropractic care. But it is reassuring to know that I haven't made the decision on blind faith; I have researched the problem from all angles and come up with the best solution for me and my health.

So whether it is advice from your doctor, your personal trainer, your naturopath or even your chiropractor, don't be afraid to get a second opinion or to research the other side of the story. It may just hold the exact solution you are looking for to get your health back on track.

The challenge: Find one problem that you have been having, or one thing you have been doing that just hasn't sat right with you and in the next 21 days go and gather some more information. Perhaps get a second opinion, perhaps seek the alternate view.

85. Finding resources

Where do you find out about health information? I mean really think about it: where have you learnt most of the health stuff you know? When you truly consider this, you will realise that much of it came from newspapers, TV, advertising, friends/family and the Internet. Are these really the sources you want to rely on for your health? Most people do more thorough research into buying a car than they do into how to look after their bodies.

We all know that papers and TV are more interested nowadays in a good story than they are in an honest story or an accurate story. In fact most of the people writing those articles and creating that TV content will have no health qualifications whatsoever and will get most of their information from commercial press releases, advertisers and special interest groups. Hardly sounds like a recipe for unbiased, accurate advice.

Advertising also has obvious flaws. Everyone wants to claim their product is the best, the healthiest, the tastiest. Ads are designed to sell products – not to be truthful and accurate.

We all know that the Internet can be very hit and miss. There is lots of great stuff on there but there is also lots of dribble. Knowing which sites are truthful and accurate can be very difficult.

What about your friends and family? Well, research shows that over 80per cent of Australians have some sort of chronic disease. In fact our rates of lifestyle diseases are getting higher and higher every year. Are these really the people you want to rely on for your health information?

So where should you get your information from?

There a number of good, healthy resources you can look at. Of course, there is my website www.drbretthill.com, but that is just one of many great resources. A couple of websites that I have used extensively over the years are www.mercola.com (lots of general health and wellness info and research) and www.crossfit.com (great functional fitness content). I also have lots of excellent books that I have read and recommend on my Amazon list (http://astore.amazon.com/drbretthillco-20). I am also fortunate to have a lot of colleagues and acquaintances who spend their lives researching and learning about health, and share that with me one-on-one and in seminars. People like Dr Damian Kristof (www.DamianKristof.com), Dr James Chestnut (www.wellnessandprevention.com) and my trainer Duncan Maxwell (www.energyclinic.net) have been instrumental in helping me develop my knowledge and philosophy. The key for you, though, is to actively find your own resources that you know and trust. Use ones that have been recommended to you by your healthcare provider or a learned friend. Check the facts and research to see that they are to be trusted, and always seek to get a couple of different points of view... because if you just rely on the information that you are being spoon-fed through the TV, Internet and your friends, then chances are, you are entrusting your health to a sales rep and a marketing guru.

The challenge: In the next 21 days find one resource that you didn't know existed before that you can trust. Repeat this challenge regularly for the rest of your life as information changes all the time and new sources constantly become available.

86. Be congruent and honest

There is no better way to stress out your body than not being honest. And it doesn't matter whether we are talking about being honest with others or with yourself.

Not being honest with others is a sure fire way to a stressed out body. Even if you don't have to go through all the stress of being caught out, you will have the tension of maintaining your lie over time not to mention the worry about the possibility of getting caught out.

The lies that we tell to ourselves are probably even worse. We might be telling ourselves that we eat 'healthily' or that we 'eat OK' when the truth is in another category altogether. These lies might not seem like much at the time, but built up over a lifetime they can lead to a seriously poor lifestyle and often serious disease.

I see it in my practice and with my wellness coaching clients all the time. People are desperately trying to find that miracle cure to their problems and looking everywhere, when the truth is right there in front of them – if only they would stop lying to themselves and allow themselves to see it!

Another lie is to do things that are not congruent with your core values. Whenever you are doing an activity that is does not sit well with your core values, be it the work you do, the way you treat people or the food you eat, you are in effect lying to yourself. You are telling yourself that it is 'OK' when deep down you realise it is not, and it is causing you to be conflicted and stressed.

So be honest with others and even more importantly be honest and congruent with yourself and you will not only be happier but also much less stressed.

The challenge: Find one thing that you have been doing that is not honest or congruent and in the next 21 days find a better way to do it. Repeat this challenge as many times as it takes until you are being honest and congruent in all aspects of your life.

87. Maintain your power

Wellness is all about taking back control of your health. So often in our modern society we have decided to palm off that responsibility to someone else.

It might be your doctor, your spouse, your mum, your TV or even society in general – we have decided that someone else gets to influence the decisions we make around our health, and more often than not, it is harming us.

Think about the last health decision you had to make. Did you really make it yourself, or did you just think you did? Did you weight up the pros and cons? Did you get a few different opinions? Did you do your own research? Did you actively go out and look for a differing opinion? Did you ask yourself whether the remedy felt right for you? Or did you just do it because your doctor said so, or because your wife nagged you, or because it is the way it has always been done?

It's OK if you are following a leader – that is your choice. But are you really happy with the results? Are you as healthy, as energetic, as vibrant as you want to be? Are you a healthy weight? Are you strong? Are you flexible? Are you emotionally stable?

If the answer is no to any or all of these things, then perhaps it is time to start doing things differently. Perhaps it is time to start making your own decisions (and yes, perhaps even your own mistakes). Perhaps it is time to remember that it is your body, and you have the right to look after it in any way that you see fit.

Start taking back your personal power when it comes to your health. Start making your own healthcare decisions, start asking the tough questions, and remember that no matter how many letters they have after their name, a doctor is only giving you advice. It is your right to decide whether you take it or leave it, and no one can ever take that away from you.

The challenge: Find one decision in your life that you have been allowing someone else to make for you and for the next 21 days take back the power. Repeat this challenge as many times as it takes until you own all your life decisions.

88. Minimize chlorine

Many people don't like drinking tap water because of the taste, especially in my home town of Adelaide where the chlorine taste is pretty strong. But the real reason not to drink the tap water may be your health.

Have you ever wondered what effect chlorine has on your body? Chlorine is present in the water because it is good for killing bacteria and so helps to remove diseases from the water supply. Unfortunately, unlike your immune system, chlorine is unable to differentiate between beneficial and unhealthy bacteria. This means that chlorine is one of the major causes of the loss of Probiotics in our body, which are very important for digestive health. Chlorine has also been shown to create free radicals which may increase vulnerability to cancers, increase ageing, destroy essential fatty acids and hinder cholesterol metabolism. The Environmental Protection Agency (EPA) in America also states that 'breathing small amounts of chlorine for short periods of time adversely affects the human respiratory system. Human health effects associated with breathing or otherwise consuming small amounts of chlorine over long periods of time are not known'.

Not only that, but chlorine reacts with organic material in our water to create DBPs (disinfection byproducts). These DBPs may be up to 10,000 times more toxic than chlorine and even worse than other water additives such as fluoride, and the levels of these in our water are closely regulated. In fact the EPA has recommended that the level of these chemicals is zero. Unfortunately though, rather than eliminating these dangerous chemicals, our authorities have decided that a certain level is acceptable. Over the years the acceptable levels around the world have been gradually decreased as the true toxicity of these chemicals has been realised.

One of the worst of these DBPs is Trihalomethanes (THMs), which have been linked to reproductive problems and miscarriages, and have even been shown to increase the risk of bladder and rectal cancer.

It's not just the chlorine in your drinking water either. One study has suggested that chlorine exposure whilst swimming accounts for approximately 94per cent of the cancer risk associated with THMs. In particular, studies have shown swimming in chlorinated water to increase the risk of melanoma. Not only are CBPs swallowed by swimmers, they are also absorbed via the skin and breathed in in the air around swimming pools (especially indoor ones where these chemicals concentrate). We are also exposed to chlorine via many other sources including chlorine byproducts released into the air by dishwashers and released into the air from industrial sources.

The challenge: For the next 21 days find one way to reduce your exposure to chlorine, be it filtering your water, finding an alternative water source or swimming in an outdoor pool – or even better, saltwater pool or ocean!

89. Reduce household toxins

We all know that our houses are full of toxic chemicals. Be they cleaning chemicals, bug sprays, detergents, personal care products, paints or garden sprays, they can contain some pretty nasty chemicals. So why doesn't it bother us?

Many people just assume that if they are allowed to be on our shelves, then they have been tested and shown to be safe. The reality is that many of these chemicals have been shown to be harmful on their own. Chemicals such as phthalates, heavy metals and pesticides have been linked to everything from cancers and nerve damage to miscarriages and birth defects. And that is just what they can do on their own – we have no idea how harmful they may be in combination. You see, we tend to test all of these chemicals in isolation, but the reality of your average household is that you have an accumulation of many different chemicals. Whilst your body may be clever enough to deal with one of these alone, the cumulative effect may be way more than your body can handle.

So how can we cut down on these chemicals?

There are many products on the market now that can help you reduce the chemical load in your household, and of course there are some old fashioned remedies that will help as well. Things like lemon juice, vinegar and baking soda can be used in place of cleaning chemicals, and the Enjo range of cleaning products can help you to clean many surfaces without any cleaning products at all. Understanding the principles of organic gardening and companion planting can help you to greatly reduce the need for chemicals in the garden. And don't worry, you don't have to throw out all those personal care products and become a long-haired hippy just yet (unless you want to). There are plenty of products on the market right now that can help you do the same job, or even better, as your favourite old chemical cocktail.

So start reading the packets of your everyday household products (some of the names alone will be enough to scare you) and chuck out those nasty chemicals!

The challenge: Find one household toxin in your home and in the next 21 days replace it with a healthy alternative. Repeat this challenge as many times as it takes until you no longer have these harmful toxins in your home.

90. Drink bottles and containers

You surely must have heard all the noise in recent times around the chemicals in our plastics. Research is pouring in showing that the petrochemicals in our plastic bottles, tin liners and clingwrap has been leaching out and infesting our food. In fact some countries are presently trying to ban these compounds. The concern is the effect these chemicals have been shown to have on the hormone systems of our bodies. The chemicals that have been singled out at this stage are Phthalates and Bisphenol A (BPA). They have been linked with erectile dysfunction, breast cancer, reproductive system cancers infertility, endometriosis and polycystic ovaries, just to name a few.

What to look out for:

Bisphenol A (BPA), usually found in hard plastics including baby drinking bottles, children's mugs, lining of tin cans and sports bottles. Look out for the 07 symbol to indicate products containing this dangerous compound.

Phthalates, found not only in our food but in plastic furniture, perfumes, make-up, liquid soaps, the plastic lining of your dishwasher and even the coatings on medications. Look out for the 01 symbol.

Many manufacturers are now cottoning on to people's concerns and creating BPA-free plastic bottles. The concern is that these bottles are replacing one petrochemical with a huge long name with another and that potentially we may be going through these exact same problems all over again in a few years or decades.

The Challenge: In the next 21 days find yourself some good solid glass containers with BPA-free lids and be sure in the knowledge that it is inert and safe. And don't worry: a good solid glass container really is hard to break. If you can find one with nice neoprene holder it will be even more unbreakable.

91. Go barefoot

Whenever I go for a personal training session at my gym, my trainer insists that I take my shoes off – and for good reason.

Not only does it protect his precious padded floors, but it provides benefits for me as well. You see, we didn't always wear padded shoes with NASA technology in the sole and dead flat bottoms, and walk around on perfectly smooth floors. In fact, modern shoes may be so 'good' they are making your feet lazy, weak and prone to injury.

The truth is our bodies need movement and our feet are no exception. Exercising with no shoes enables your foot to go through a larger range of motion. It also helps to strengthen the muscles in and around the foot because they are activated a lot more without the shoes taking up the slack.

There is also a neurological reason for going barefoot. With your shoes off you will fire more of the nerve endings (proprioception) in your feet that tell your brain where your body is in space. This is important not just for improving your balance and coordination but also because of the effect it has on your brain. After your spine, your feet are one of the most important sources of this important feedback which has been likened to a windmill which drives the power station of your brain by researchers.

There are of course a few things you need to consider before you head off footloose and fancy free. Some places are inappropriate to be barefoot. Your local gym probably won't appreciate it if you are running barefoot on their treadmill or putting your sweaty feet on their weights machines. You should also be aware of your environment. Things like broken glass and even something as simple as a stray twig can do serious damage to a bare foot.

If it just isn't practical to go barefoot though there are still plenty of options. There are a whole series of shoes on the market now that let your feet move in a much more natural manner. There are a few runners specifically designed to mimic barefoot training and almost all of the martial arts shoes will do the trick too. In fact even that good old Aussie icon the Dunlop Volley can be a great shoe to allow much more freedom and movement of your feet without the massive heel lift. I like to call these shoes 'functional' shoes

Finally some conditions will prohibit barefoot exercising, for instance a diabetic with limited foot sensation may cause serious damage before they even notice a problem. So as always consult your health care professional.

The challenge: Once a week for the next 7 weeks do your exercise routine without shoes or with functional shoes. Repeat this challenge as many times as it takes until you are wearing no shoes wherever practical and 'functional' shoes when it's not.

92. Get in control of your money

Money is definitely one of the biggest stressors for many, many people. The biggest problem most people have in regards to their money is that they just bury their heads in the sand. It all just seems too hard, so they avoid stressing about their money problems by ignoring them completely. Unfortunately this never works. Because of the nature of money and expenses, you are forced to confront these fears every day whether you want to or not, and the more you try and ignore them the bigger the problem becomes.

The key to reducing your money fears is to get informed.

1. Find out how much money you have. It is amazing how many people have money in all different spots and debt in even more places and just don't realise what their actual financial position is. The truth is less stressful than not knowing, because at least once you know, you can start to manage it.

2. Find out how much you make. Sounds simple doesn't it, but you would be surprised how many people don't actually know how much they take home each week after tax. Especially those that don't have a fixed salary. If this is you, then work it out over three months and average it to get a good picture.

3. Find out how much you spend. People always think of a budget as being boring and restrictive but this doesn't need to be the case. You can allow room in your budget for splurging on whatever you love splurging on. The difference now will be that you can do it guilt-free because you know you can afford it.

4. Find out what possible solutions there are to your budgetary issues. So often people who have debt issues,

cash flow issues and budgeting issues are too scared to do anything about it. The best thing you can do is speak to people in the know or read knowledgeable resources and you will be amazed that the solutions aren't as scary as you thought. When I was a boy, my parents bought me *Rich Dad, Poor Dad* by Robert Kiyosaki and I still think it is a great way to start.

So when it comes to money and stress, stop sticking your head in the sand. Get yourself informed about your true status and real solutions, and you will be amazed at how much the reduced stress influences your everyday life and health.

The challenge: In the next 21 days find out exactly how much money you have, how much money you make, how much money you spend and where you spend it. Once you have all this information start searching for ways you can do it better. Repeat this challenge on a regular basis (at least once a year).

93. Healthy rewards

I always find it strange that people will work so hard at their diet or so hard at their exercise regime and decide they need a reward – only to have that reward undo some (if not all) of the hard work they have just done. They say to themselves, 'I have worked really hard, I deserve this special treat'. It is especially concerning when people start doing the same thing for their kids.

Why would people think that for working so hard to get healthy, they deserve to have all that hard work undone? Even worse, why would people think it is a good idea to teach themselves and their families that junk foods or unhealthy behaviour are special treats and should be associated with rewards and fun?

Don't get me wrong: I am as prone to guilty snacks or slip-ups as anyone. The difference is, I never consider it a reward or a gift for my body. I always understand that whilst a big piece of cake isn't the end of the world, it isn't something to be celebrating either. The problem with unhealthy foods as a reward is that it teaches your body bad habits. Your body (and your mind) will associate unhealthy choices with celebrating, being happy and feeling good. So next time you are feeling a bit down guess what is going to happen? This is true tenfold for kids.

When I really want to reward myself, I do it by finding something that I really love – often something that I don't always do or have – that is healthy, and enjoying that. By doing so I know that not only am I rewarding my good behaviour and celebrating my successes in the short term, but in the long term as well.

So next time you feel like a tasty reward, why not choose a punnet of blueberries or strawberries rather than a bag of lollies? Why not your favourite active pastime (like golf or shopping) rather than slobbing around on the couch? You will not only enjoy the riches today, you will enjoy the benefits tomorrow as well!

The challenge: For the next 21 days replace one of your regular unhealthy 'rewards' with a healthy alternative. Repeat this challenge as many times as it takes until you are only rewarding yourself with healthy stuff (except for the very rare exception).

94. Maintain your curiosity

Curiosity may have killed the cat but it is a lack of curiosity that kills a human. Well, perhaps that is a little extreme, but you get the idea. It is important for us to remain curious so that we can be open to the changes we need to make in order to keep ourselves in shape.

So often we make health choices based on old information. What we were taught at school, what our doctor was taught at school, what our parents did, what our neighbours parents did, well you get the idea. If we don't challenge the status quo, if we don't do different things, then how can we expect to get different results? And we certainly need to get different results. You only need to look around you to see that as a society we are sicker than ever and not due to germs, not due to genes, not even due to bad luck – but due to our lifestyles. So now is the time to get curious, to start asking those tricky questions. Start challenging what you do on a day-to-day basis and whether it is contributing to your health or detracting from it.

What if all this stuff I have been doing is wrong? What if the food pyramid isn't accurate? What if half an hour of walking five days a week isn't really all my body requires? What if the way I perceive the world isn't how it really is? Ask yourself these and the million other little questions that will start to spring into your head when you start to take a curious approach to life, and you will get some interesting answers.

In life it is easy to be stagnant, to settle, to get in a rut. The only way to get out of it is to start asking great questions. The answers may just save your life (or at least your health)!

The challenge: For one day this week as you go through your day challenge everything. Have a really critical look at every decision you make along your way from the way you go to work to the way you talk to what you eat to how you dress. All day ask yourself the question 'what if...' repeat this challenge as many times as it takes until you are making curiosity a regular habit.

95. Running right

You don't need anyone to teach you how to run, right? Well, that's what I thought until recently, when I realised that for most of the first 30 years of my life I have been doing it wrong. It had never made sense to me that running was considered such an unhealthy activity in terms of the effects of the impact on your body, or that so many people were getting injuries just from running. After all, once upon a time it was the only way we could get around. Did the Kalahari bushmen suffer from knee degeneration or Iliotibial band syndrome? Somehow I think not.

Chances are that when I started out running around barefoot as a kid I was doing it properly, but over time my environment (and my shoes) have trained me to do it differently. You see, when we run in our modern shoes on flat roads – or even worse, treadmills – we tend to get lazy with our running. We tend to strike the ground with our heels first, stand upright, don't lift our feet very far off of the ground, and for many people, this leads to poor posture.

Do me a favour. Take off your shoes and go run around outside on the grass – or even better, watch a bunch of kids running around barefoot. Look really closely. Which part of their foot hits the ground first?

You will find that it is the mid-foot (essentially the ball of the foot, or a spot just behind the ball). This is a natural running style. It allows the heel to be lowered more softly onto the ground and drastically reduces the impact of the run. Now if you have good posture when you run and you stand up nice and straight with your gluteals (bum) and your abs engaged and your shoulders back, you will soon realise that in order to land on your mid-foot, you will have to lean forward.

Leaning forward also means that your centre of gravity is in front of your feet. The combination of not striking with your heels (after all, how do you slow down going down a hill?) and leaning forward leads to a much more natural run with greater speed and less effort as well. Sounds too good to be true, doesn't it? Well, that's what I thought until I started doing it. Now I can do exactly the same run as I did before, and I do it easier, faster and have less tiredness and fatigue afterwards.

So if I can't have my traditional runners, what shoes should I wear?

Well, some people have started running with no shoes at all, but for most of us using your average roads and paths, that is a bit extreme. Fortunately there is a whole swag of shoes coming onto the market now that are designed specifically for this purpose. There are Newton runners, Nike Frees and Vibram Five Fingers, just to name a few. Even the good old Dunlop volleys are probably better than what you are wearing now for most people.

The challenge: Analyse your running technique (there is more to it than you think) and do one run with either no shoes or shoes that encourage a mid-foot strike.

96. Eat less un-fermented soy

Soy is a health food, right?

Well, research would pretty comprehensively suggest that it's not. So why is there still so much confusion? And why is soy still so popular? So popular, in fact, that it has been estimated that Soybeans form 10per cent of the total calories ingested in the United States. Soy is present in everything from the obvious (soy milk, soy cheese and soy meat replacements) to the hidden (many processed foods).

It all started in 1999 when the FDA (food and drug adminis-tration) in America approved a health claim that a high soy diet reduced heart disease. Soy was really one of the first foods to get on the health marketing band wagon. A few studies suggested that soy may help to reduce heart disease and the PR machine kicked in. All of a sudden soy was the new 'it' product and everyone was jumping on the trend. Soy is marketed so well that even now, when there are so many studies suggesting otherwise, it is still considered by the general population to be a healthy product.

So what's wrong with soy?

There are three major problems with the way we now consume soy. We eat it in large quantities, it is highly processed and it is often unfermented.

Processed unfermented soy has high levels of 'anti-nutrients' and toxins that are naturally present in soy beans as well as toxic residues created by the processing. As a result, intake of soy has been linked to cancer, reproductive disorders, brain damage and thyroid problems (including weight gain, loss of libido and lethargy). Isoflavones in the soy are also phytoestrogens meaning that they mimic the action of oestrogen in the body and can adversely affect your hormone balance, especially in kids. Soy oil (like most vegetable oils) is also high in Omega 6 fatty acids, which leads to an unhealthy fat balance.

Most soy is also genetically modified. This is a concern for two reasons. One, it is pretty strongly linked to allergies. In fact soy is now the second most common food allergy in America behind peanuts. Secondly, the reason it is genetically modified is so that it isn't killed by herbicides. That means that they have designed it so that they can spray it with herbicides that would usually kill it – and that's why GM soy crops are sprayed 86per cent more than non-GM crops.

Soy is also 'hidden' in many foods, especially in the form of oil. If you check the ingredients list on many of the processed foods you find in the supermarket, you will find soy oil and soy proteins are really common ingredients.

The exception to the rule in terms of soy products is the traditionally fermented varieties. Foods like Tempeh and Miso and traditionally fermented soy sauce are actually quite healthy in small doses. The fermentation process reduces the toxins in the soy and reduces the levels of the oestrogenic chemicals.

The challenge: Start checking your food labels for unfermented soy products. For the next 21 days replace one unfermented soy containing food with a non-soy alternative.

97. Avoid fluoride

For most Australians, when you are drinking your tap water, you are really taking medication. Yes that's right: our water has been medicated by the addition of fluoride. But that's OK because it's good for our teeth, right?

Well, perhaps not. Studies show that there is little or no difference in rates of tooth decay in communities where the water is fluoridated. In fact the dental costs are actually higher due to the dental fluorosis which is a side-effect of this medication. It is interesting to note that in 2009, Tasmania – the first state to introduce fluoride into the drinking water (and with an 83per cent fluoridation rate, compared to Queensland's 54per cent) – also has the highest rates of tooth decay.

We are often shown graphs of the reduction in dental decay since the introduction of fluoride in the 1970s. What we are not told, however, is that this reduction has also occurred in countries that do not fluoridate their water. Or that in Finland and Germany the decay rates have remained stable or continued to decline after water fluoridation was removed. In fact many nations including France, Austria, Denmark, Iceland, Italy, Japan, The Netherlands, Norway, Sweden and Switzerland and the UK either do not fluoridate or have very low rates of water fluoridation.

Dental fluorosis leads to black or brown stains, cracking, pitting and even mottling of dental enamel. Sounds kind of like what we were trying to prevent, right? The critical period of fluoride exposure for fluorosis is from 1 to 4 years of age which really highlights the key issue of mass medication. It doesn't take into account the differing needs of different members of the population. Not only do these kids not need fluoride at this age, but they are more susceptible to its adverse effects due to the relatively high intake compared to their relatively smaller body size. In fact in 2006 the American Dental Association warned parents not to use fluoridated water in their baby formulas.

Fluoride can be naturally present in water supplies in the form of calcium fluoride, however this is not the fluoride that is added to our water supply. Ninety per cent of what is added to our water is solicofluoride, which is up to 85 times more toxic than the naturally occurring form. These unnatural fluorides are also not easily eliminated from the body like the natural forms, meaning that the levels build up over time.

So why do we use unnatural fluorides then? The reason is that it is a cheap by product of phosphate fertiliser, aluminium and steel production and has the added bonus of ridding that industry of a dangerous toxin it would otherwise have to pay to safely dispose of. In fact the original, poorly designed studies that are still used to justify water fluoridation are widely believed to have had links to these very industries.

So just how bad is fluoride? Well, the problem is, we don't really know. There have not been enough high quality studies into the health effects of fluoridation to give a conclusive answer. There are however studies showing links between fluoridation and poor thyroid function, arthritis, bone cancer, lower IQ and osteoporosis. So given the limited benefits and the known risks, I would definitely avoid this mass medication campaign.

People also often don't realise that a simple carbon filter will not remove fluoride. So if you live in an area with a fluoridated water supply (fortunately I don't) you should either use a reverse osmosis water filter (which removes 65-95per cent of the fluoride) or distil all your water. And don't forget to treat the water you bathe and shower in and also the water you use to wash your fruits and veggies.

The Challenge: Either source water that is clean and untreated, or purchase a good quality water purification system to remove these unneeded medications from your water supply.

So you finally made it to the end...

Have you started Eating The Elephant? Or have you just read through the whole book and not actually DONE anything? This book is a great **resource** and can be a fantastic **resource** for creating significant change in your health and your life, BUT it won't do it by itself and it certainly won't do it if you leave it gathering dust on the bookshelf. And please don't try and tell me that there are no suitable challenges, or that they are all too hard or not applicable. I mean honestly – if you can't find a suitable challenge in the pages of this book, then you are just not trying!

In the words of legendary AFL coach John Kennedy Senior, "At least DO SOMETHING! DO! Don't think, don't hope, do! At least you can come off and say... 'At least I did something'.

About the Author

Dr Brett Hill is a wellness expert, chiropractor and health author. He regularly appears on TV, radio and in print, and his media appearances, seminars, coaching and consulting have inspired thousands of people over the last decade to live a long, happy, healthy life full of energy and vitality.

In his early 20s, Dr Brett realised that it was time to make a change; something had to give. Over the course of the next decade he gradually turned his life around. He started getting regular chiropractic care, cleaned up his diet, started exercising well and in the process he learnt what it takes to make real life-long changes to lifestyle and health.

In the process Dr Brett has been able to share his journey with his fabulous wife Rebecca and now their two gorgeous children Tom and Charlotte, who have inspired Dr Brett to take his message to the world in order to create a healthier environment for his family to thrive in.

Dr Brett's websites, articles, videos, media appearances and books have inspired people all over the world to make drastic changes for the better in their life and their health.

Highlights from Dr Brett's dynamic career include:

- Editorial in publications as diverse as The Adelaide Magazine, Men's Health and The Borneo Post and The Advertiser newspaper.
- Online editorial on NineMSN, AdelaideNow and more
- Radio appearances on ABC, 5AA, FreshFM, Fresh 102.3 and others
- TV appearances on Channel Seven and Channel Nine
- Wellness seminars including Queensland's Dynamic Growth Congress, corporations, councils and more
- Launching popular health resource www.drbretthill.com

and monthly newsletter
- His successful chiropractic and wellness coaching practice in Linden Park, South Australia

Dr Hill is a Doctor of Chiropractic and holds a Bachelor of Health Science (The University of Adelaide) and Masters of Chiropractic (Macquarie University, NSW) and is President of the Chiropractors Association of Australia (SA).

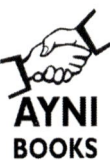

AYNI
BOOKS

Ayni Books publishes complementary and alternative approaches to health, healing and well-being, following a holistic model.